Living Longer, Living Better

Exploring the Heart-Mind Connection

Previous books by the author:

Drugs for the Heart, 7th Edition
Lionel H. Opie and Bernard J. Gersh
(Saunders, 2008)

Heart Physiology: From Cell to Circulation, 4th Edition
Lionel H. Opie
(Lippincott, Williams & Wilkins, 2004)

Cardiology at the Limits, 10th edition
Co-edited by Lionel H. Opie

Diabetes at the Limits, 3rd edition
Co-edited by Lionel H. Opie

Living Longer, Living Better
Exploring the Heart-Mind Connection

Lionel H. Opie

OXFORD
UNIVERSITY PRESS

OXFORD
UNIVERSITY PRESS

Great Clarendon Street, Oxford ox2 6dp

Oxford University Press is a department of the University of Oxford.
It furthers the University's objective of excellence in research, scholarship, and education by publishing worldwide in

Oxford New York

Auckland Cape Town Dar es Salaam Hong Kong Karachi
Kuala Lumpur Madrid Melbourne Mexico City Nairobi
New Delhi Shanghai Taipei Toronto

With offices in

Argentina Austria Brazil Chile Czech Republic France Greece
Guatemala Hungary Italy Japan Poland Portugal Singapore
South Korea Switzerland Thailand Turkey Ukraine Vietnam

Published in the United States
by Oxford University Press Inc., New York

First published 2011

British Library Cataloguing-in-Publication Data
Data available

Library of Congress Cataloging-in-Publication Data

Typeset by Glyph International, Bangalore, India
Printed in Great Britain
on acid-free paper by
Clays Ltd, St Ives plc

ISBN 978–0–19–852567–7

10 9 8 7 6 5 4 3 2 1

Whilst every effort has been made to ensure that the contents of this book are as complete, accurate and-up-to-date as possible at the date of writing. Oxford University Press is not able to give any guarantee or assurance that such is the case. Readers are urged to take appropriately qualified medical advice in all cases. The information in this book is intended to be useful to the general reader, but should not be used as a means of self-diagnosis or for the prescription of medication.

Foreword

by a leading international Health and Lifestyle Scientist

Our destinies are sometimes determined by seemingly mystical circumstances.

On the afternoon of my 17th Birthday on July 2nd 1966, cardiac surgeon, Dr Adrian Kantrowitz was preparing to perform the world's first human heart transplant at the Maimonides Hospital in Brooklyn, New York. But the heart of the donor would cease beating minutes before the operation could begin, ending Kantrowitz's brush with immortality.

Instead on the night of 3rd December 1967, Professor Christiaan Barnard performed the world's first successful human heart transplant at Groote Schuur Hospital in Cape Town, South Africa. This set in motion a series of events, one consequence of which was the invitation from my mentor, friend and hero, Lionel Opie, to write the foreword for this book. There are few assignments that could fill me with greater pleasure.

Professor Barnard's pioneering operation profoundly influenced both our lives. In Lionel's case the operation encouraged his return from London to his alma mater, the University of Cape Town, to establish a laboratory for the study of the heart, its biology and diseases. The operation also inspired me, in my youthful uncertainty, to study medicine in Cape Town. Without that first heart transplant, neither Lionel, the lecturer, nor I, the student, would have been at Groote Schuur Hospital on that afternoon in September 1972 when Lionel presented his lecture on heat stroke to our group of fifth year medical students. Lionel, the new appointee in the Department of Medicine, had been allocated this orphan lecture that none other wished; I had a special interest in heat stroke since it addressed sport and medicine, the source of my enduring intellectual passion.

Lionel's lecture was quite unlike anything I had ever heard – he transformed the orphan into a regal beauty. The lecture came not from the textbook, but from a careful analysis of the published literature including all its certainties and doubts. Lionel presented his own conclusions and detailed the logic by which he had arrived at that wisdom. I was utterly mesmerized. It was plain that the lecture was the product of a unique intellect. So inspired, three years later I began my career as a medical scientist in his heart laboratory. So began a relationship now approaching its fifth decade that has been one of the enduring joys of my life. Perhaps I may be granted the presumption that I am qualified to write the truth about my long-time friend and inspiration.

Lionel is quite evidently one of the very finest scientists ever produced by South Africa. He belongs also to a select group of the world's very best scientific communicators. His eminence arises from his relentless, single-minded pursuit of new knowledge and his ability to synthesize and to present all information, from the simplest to the most complex, better than anyone I know or have ever heard. He is driven by a tireless search for perfection – perfection in analysis, in logic, in interpretation, in understanding and, not least, in presentation.

He is recognized globally for his publications on the biology and pharmacology of the heart. His books are the universal standard. They are the product of 50 years of focused study by an uncommon intellect, honed to perfection and communicated with uncommon skills. They achieve their supreme status because they are complete – nothing important is missing. Despite their completeness they radiate simplicity – the simplicity of concealed truths available to us all but which are assembled into a complete wisdom only by those select few with a unique combination of abilities.

When Lionel turned his attention to the science of healthy living, I knew that he would produce something extraordinary, better than anything ever before attempted or achieved. And so it has happened. In *Heart and Mind*, Lionel has produced the new standard. It is a masterpiece. The book can be described in one word – perfect. It is perfect because it presents the complete scientific evidence, critically analyzed by the world's most qualified mind, clearly, concisely and without condescension. Here there is no place for the writing method of the health gurus whose unsubstantiated personal beliefs are more usually fuelled by narcissism and personal interest than by the search for eternal truths.

As I read each page for the first time, I was filled with the same awe and wonder that I experience each time I read any of Lionel's work. The overwhelming impression is the simple beauty of the prose he constructs - its clarity, rhythm and urgency, complimented by his trademark line diagrams when words alone are not enough.

By writing this book Lionel properly exposes his genius to a lay audience for the first time. I know of no one who understands the heart more completely or who can express himself with greater effect to any audience than can Lionel. I also know of now other whose opinion on the heart I would trust with greater certainty.

For those who wish to know the truth of this matter, this is the book.

Professor Timothy Noakes OMS, MD, DSc
Discovery Health Professor of Exercise and Sports Science,
Department of Human Biology,
University of Cape Town and Sports Science Institute of
South Africa,
Cape Town, South Africa.

Foreword

by a leading Oxford Cardiologist

Heart disease is the number one killer in the Western World, while dementia, or the loss of one's mind, is one of the leading causes of disability. In an ever ageing society, both are expected to take an even greater toll on coming generations. We all know someone affected by one of these two great modern scourges. And most of us worry whether heart disease or dementia will one day – soon or in the more distant future – strike ourselves, robbing us of precious life years and/or their quality. But what can we do to counter the threat, and where do we get authoritative advice we can trust? *The Heart-Mind Connection*, a book written by one of the greatest Cardiologists of all times, Professor Lionel Opie, achieves exactly that.

I first came across the name Lionel Opie when I started a lifelong interest in cardiac research as a postdoc at Harvard Medical School in 1985. When exploring the literature, his name seemed to pop up everywhere. I remember asking my professor at the time – who is this Mr. Opie? The answer still sticks in my mind today – "Professor Opie, young fellow, is one of the real giants of cardiovascular science". When I met Lionel for the first time many years later, I was deeply impressed by his unique combination of scientific excellence and rigour, deep intellectual insight into the inner works of the cardiovascular system, all achieved with the humility of a decent "down-to-earth" researcher, who simply wants to get to the bottom of the scientific truth. In the world of Cardiology, when Lionel speaks, his colleagues listen! Professor Opie has made his scientific impact through countless important research articles, but here he has done something very few scientists of his calibre have attempted before – to take his lifetime of experience and turn it into a textbook written for a much wider audience – the so-called "educated lay person". In this book, he manages to apply the same rigorous scientific principles that characterise his research articles to a more general format, one easily accessible to the non-specialist. In so doing, he has given a broad readership the chance to benefit from his wisdom. And where scientific data are sparse or non-existent, he is not shy to provide his firm opinion, based on his wealth of experience.

In eight chapters, Professor Opie sets out his vision of how the heart and mind connect. Chapter one takes us through the origins of human life and explains how body responses originally designed as adaptive and life saving can become detrimental in the modern world. Chapter two explains the elements contributing to a healthy heart and mind, and where things can go wrong. In chapter three, clear and detailed advice is given on what is required for a healthy lifestyle. In my clinical Cardiology practice, patients often ask me about what exactly their diet should look like – I am glad I can now refer them to Chapter four of this book, which deals with all such diet related issues, from the different kinds of fat and their qualities, advice on varied foods such as nuts and avocados, to the detailed assessment of the different diet options such as Mediterranean (the ideal diet), Atkins, etc. In Chapter five, Professor Opie takes us through a range of current medical myths and promises, such as the failure of vitamin supplements, the role of coffee and tea, or the interesting and deceptively simple question of how much water we should drink. Expect clear and authoritative answers! The final three Chapters explore questions of the mind, ranging from the medical risk factors affecting the brain, through strategies for preservation of cognitive function and memory. The book culminates in a thorough analysis of what connects the heart with the mind, exploring how the state of "*mindfulness*" can be achieved and how we can take charge of controlling stress in life – meditation, passion and play are some of the recommendations, and you can be sure Professor Opie excels at those too! Take it all in, and don't miss the chance to learn about important and truly life changing measures.

The Heart-Mind Connection provides us with the answers to the burning questions we have about living a longer, better and generally more positive and productive life, and it puts the scientific evidence in perspective with a holistic view. Reading this book and digesting all its masterful wisdom is a must!

Professor Stefan Neubauer MD, FRCP, FACC, FMedSci
Professor of Cardiovascular Medicine,
Department of Cardiovascular Medicine,
University of Oxford, UK

Contents

Contributors

Joseph Raimondo,
MSc Neurosciences (Oxon); MB, ChB (Cape Town);
Rhodes Scholar, Lincoln College
Department of Pharmacology,
Oxford University, UK

Jeannie Walker,
Medical Illustrator

Helen Moffett,
Medical Writer

Introduction

Lionel H. Opie, MD, DPhil (Oxon)

Director Emeritus, Hatter Cardiovascular Research Institute, Cape Heart Centre, Chris Barnard Building, University of Cape Town, South Africa; International Associate Editor of *Circulation*, the American Heart Association; Co-editor and founder, *Drugs for the Heart* 7th ed., 2009

Visiting Professor, Department of Cardiovascular Medicine, Stanford University, California, 1984–1998.

Honarary Professor, Hatter Institute for Cardiovascular Research, University College London.

Visiting Research Fellow, Merton College and Department of Physiology, University of Oxford, United Kingdom, 1997

This book is aimed at those who strive for optimal long-term health and maximal functioning of their hearts and minds. Today's problem for the health-conscious person is information overload—new health studies pour out almost daily from newspapers, radio stations, and television networks. Many of the reports are contradictory and often misleading. My aim is to guide readers through this morass of information. The message is that a specific number of key steps taken now will give protection from future heart disease or brain deterioration.

After reading countless original articles in scientific journals and listening to experts at international conferences, as well as keeping my ears open when patients tell me about their experiences, I have sifted through almost all of the available information with the aim of grading the validity of the evidence. Just how true are the studies? Just how compelling are the facts they claim? From the vast number of possible health promotion changes, varying from increased exercise to aspirin to green tea, and diets from Atkins to the vegetarian, only five lifestyle changes reach the status of having compelling evidence. I call these the 'big five'. (If you are curious, jump ahead to Fig. 3.1.) Following these simple steps will promote long-term health benefits for heart and mind, as well as give protection from the inroads of ageing. In addition, I will discuss how the healthy lifestyle can be aided by the correct choice of approved medications, based on my experience of over 25 years of writing and editing *Drugs for the Heart*, of which more than 150,000 copies have been sold.

How to get at the truth: relative versus absolute changes

Which of us is not bewildered by the numerous conflicting reports in the media? What we often forget is that newspapers must present health data in a simplified and sometimes sensational mode so that the paper can sell. In a similar way, television programmes extract the most extreme aspects of new information, which is then presented as a flash. But the basic, rather unexciting information often remains the same, or at best the advance is incremental rather than fundamental.

Therefore, the real aim of self-education is to gain background knowledge of solid fact, into which new information can be slotted. When assessing the significance of health information in newspapers or on television, it is essential to distinguish between relative and absolute change. For example, some years ago a report came out that hormone replacement therapy (HRT) increased heart attacks by 29% in women. That sounds prohibitively drastic. But what does that statistic really mean? Supposing a woman has no increase of risk beyond that of her age, due to her excellent lifestyle, then an increase of 29% on top of the basic 0% absolute risk is still zero. Of course it is not that simple because everyone has some risk of heart attack, but if you replace 0% by 4–6%, 29% of those small numbers is still acceptably low.

Association versus causation

Reports of new studies in the newspapers and on television often come from information gathered by association, rather than causation. An example is the large Nurses' Health Study in the United States, in which the investigators followed up the health of nurses over many years and found that nurses who had higher blood levels of vitamin E had fewer heart attacks. That result could simply be an association rather than proof that self-dosing with vitamin E improves the health of nurses and even, by implication, of women in general. For example, it could be that women taking vitamin E as an antioxidant were more intelligent and conversant with magazine articles on the benefits of antioxidants, hence being more careful with their diet and less likely to smoke.

Thus, association is not guilt, as in a court of law. In the case of vitamin E, as in every other case, it is necessary to delve into and to evaluate the controlled randomized studies that correct for lifestyle variation between the different participants. Thus in such a trial each participant would be given either the active vitamin E or a placebo (tablets or capsules looking like those of vitamin E, but not containing the active ingredient) and then the two large groups of patients have to be matched regarding age and cardiac health risks. Such a study has already been done by the research group of Dr Salim Yusuf at McMaster University in Canada. Their study showed that giving a standard dose of vitamin E continued over many years in patients at high risk for heart attacks did not improve outcome and, in fact, somewhat increased the risk of developing heart failure. Nonetheless, millions of people keep on taking vitamin E, despite such a negative outcome study.

The criteria required for proof of benefit

To have strong evidence for any therapeutic agent or lifestyle change requires, in my view, three essentials. First, there has to be *strong laboratory evidence* that the intervention works. That, for example, is the case with exercising rats that Tim Noakes, author of the foreword to this book and of the *Lore of Running*, studied in my research laboratory in Cape Town. He showed that hearts from these rats were more resistant to model heart attacks and to the irregular heart rhythm that causes sudden cardiac death in humans. Regarding omega-3 fish oils, Alexander Leaf, at the Massachusetts General Hospital of Harvard Medical School, showed in his laboratories that the omega-3 fatty acids stabilized heart cell membranes.

Secondly, there should be *population studies* to show an association. These are also called observational studies because the research workers observe certain associations without proving cause and effect. Thus those individuals who exercise more should live longer and have fewer heart attacks, as is the case. Those who have diets high in oily fish containing omega-3 fish oils should also have fewer heart attacks, as they do. Population studies lead to a hypothesis but do not provide scientific proof.

Thirdly, there must be *prospective trials*. For example, large and well-designed prospectively randomized studies must show that making the lifestyle change now improves health in the future. Thus, for example, in the case of exercise, increased intensity of exercise versus continuation of the ordinary level leads to prevention of new diabetes, which is a disease that promotes heart attacks. In the case of omega-3 capsules, when given in a well-designed trial to a large number of patients after heart attacks, the incidence of sudden cardiac death was reduced.

Often, in the course of this book, I shall refer to the difference between relative and absolute risk. Furthermore, we should constantly be asking ourselves about the level of information presented.

Examples of the threefold criteria for proof of benefit

Essential criteria	Exercise	Omega-3 fish oils
1. Laboratory evidence	Running rats have fewer heart attacks	Omega-3 fish oils prevent development of abnormal electrical currents that cause sudden cardiac death in heart attacks
2. Epidemiological evidence (observational)	Highly-trained athletes live longer	Populations with a high intake of fish oils have fewer heart attacks
3. Prospective trial evidence (randomized)	Intense exercise helps to prevent diabetes, which in turn is a major cause of heart attacks	After heart attacks, omega-3 capsules decrease sudden cardiac death (need high doses)

Laboratory data do not provide proof of efficacy, but point to the need for further human studies, first observational and then randomized.

I hope you enjoy this book and, much more importantly, learn to live well and longer.

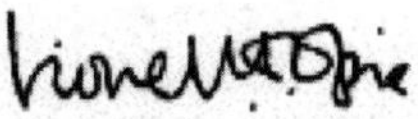

Lionel H. Opie
Cape Town, South Africa, 1 November 2010

P.S. The Mediterranean diet is not only the most healthy of all diets, but has just been immortalised by the declaration that it now belongs to the Intangible Cultural Heritage of Europe.

Chapter 1

In the Beginning

Early humans were forced to develop major protective mechanisms. They lived in semi-tropical and grassland regions, and dangerous confrontations with wild animals and natural forces such as rushing rivers were part of the everyday struggle to find food and water. These were stressful conditions, requiring fast reactions and swift running speeds in order to escape certain death (Fig. 1.1). In time, early humans developed physiological systems that made this kind of speed possible.

To help humans to run fast and respond appropriately to psychological stressors, such as acute fear, the subconscious or autonomic (which means not subject to voluntary commands) nervous system developed. This system could be automatically and subconsciously activated in response to a 'fight or flight' stimulus; for example, the rapid rise in heart rate needed to run fast in response to the stress of sighting an enemy or dangerous animal.

The nervous system has two branches. The sympathetic nervous system increases heart rate and blood pressure (BP) in response to (and thus in sympathy with) external physical or psychological stress (Fig. 1.2). Clearly, this activating system needs to be switched off at night, or when humans (whether primitive or modern-day) need to sleep or simply relax. This is when the second balancing system, which counters the activity of the sympathetic system, comes into play. It is called the parasympathetic nervous system—'para' meaning 'beside or adjacent to' (Fig. 1.3). These two systems have opposing actions: the sympathetic raises heart rate and blood pressure, and the parasympathetic decreases both, so that at night (the time of rest) the heart beats more slowly and blood pressure is lowered.

Over millions of years, these two mutually balancing nervous systems evolved to control heart rate and blood pressure, while the kidneys evolved to regulate the balance of water and salt in the blood by

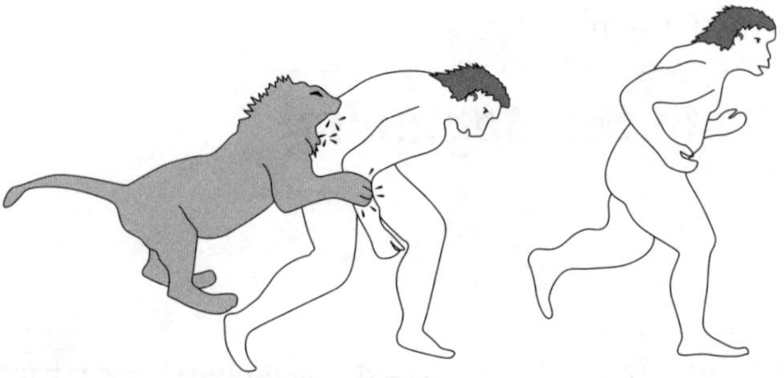

Figure 1.1 The physical stresses of primitive humans. To escape required rapid activation of the unconscious (sympathetic) nervous system (see Fig. 1.2). © Opie.

varying the composition of the urine produced, and the immune system developed to protect against the numerous tropical infective agents. Finally, these systems were able to equip early humans with enough defences against the forces of nature to allow and promote migration from the origins of humankind in East Africa to Asia, Europe, and elsewhere in Africa.

Although each of these major regulatory systems can contribute to major cardiovascular disease and problems of the heart and brain (in the circumstances in which current urban dwellers live), this book will concentrate on the interaction between the brain and the heart, and how they influence each other—for better or for worse. To start with, it's important that we understand the nervous system, how it helps us when we are threatened, and how it can overact to cause disease.

The autonomic nervous system

This system operates 24 hours a day without our conscious knowledge, but we can control its activity indirectly by means of our emotional state or by physical activity. As mentioned above, the autonomic system has two branches: first, the sympathetic nervous system, consisting of nerves running from the brain stem to the heart—to

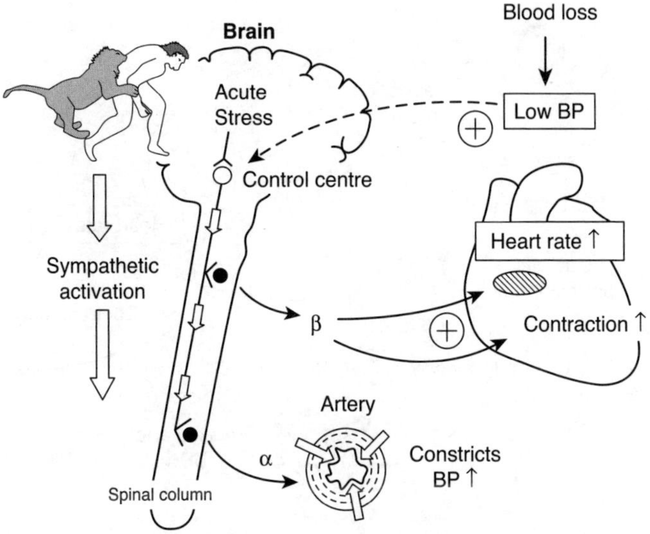

Figure 1.2 Our hearts beat faster when we are stressed: the sympathetic branch of the autonomic (subconscious) nervous system. Starting with physical or emotional stress in the conscious mind, nervous stimulation travels to the brain stem, in which the nerve control centres that govern the unconscious or autonomic nervous system are located. The sympathetic, stimulatory part of the control centre sends out an impulse that ultimately increases the heart rate and constricts the blood arteries (at bottom of figure), raising the blood pressure. The inhibitory or parasympathetic system opposes these effects (Fig. 1.3). Normally, there is a balance between the two systems, tipped towards sympathetic dominance during emotional stress or exercise, and towards parasympathetic dominance during sleep or relaxation. The sympathetic outflow runs along the spinal canal, from where further nerves convey the stimulatory impulses to the heart and arteries, where the messengers adrenaline and noradrenaline are liberated at the nerve endings. These hormones (also called epinephrine and norepinephrine in the US) act on the beta (β) receptors to make the heart beat faster and more strongly, and on the constricting alpha (α) receptors in arteries to raise the blood pressure. © Opie.

increase the heart's rate of beating, and its force of contraction—and to the arterioles (small arteries), to constrict these and thereby increase blood pressure (Fig. 1.2). While it is widely known that stress acts via this system (also called the adrenergic or the adrenaline nervous

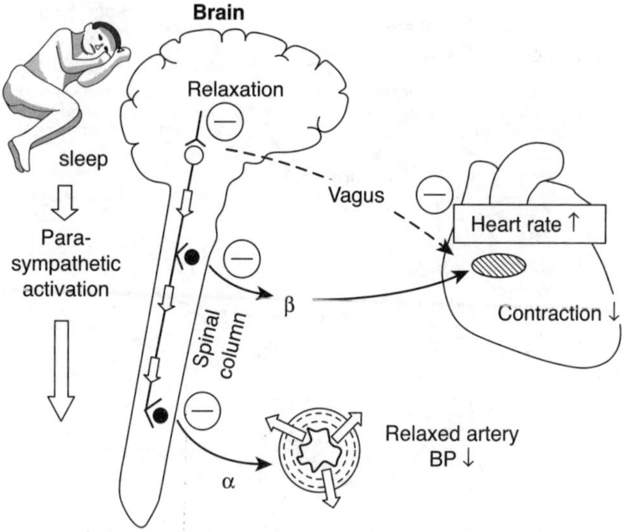

Figure 1.3 How the parasympathetic system counters the adrenaline rush. As shown in Fig. 1.2, the sympathetic stimulatory part of the control centre sends out impulses that increase the heart rate and constrict the blood arteries, raising the blood pressure. The inhibitory parasympathetic system opposes these effects. This system is also called the *vagal system* because it originates in the vagal nerve nucleus in the lower brain, and reaches the heart and small arteries (arterioles) via branches of the vagal nerve. For alpha (α) and beta (β), see legend to Fig. 1.2. © Opie.

system) to raise blood pressure and heart rate, it is less well known that the sympathetic system is balanced by the parasympathetic nervous system, which reduces heart rate and blood pressure (Table 1.1).

Why have these systems evolved? Clearly, increases in heart rate and blood pressure are required when chasing a wild animal, or when battling an opposing male for the fair hand of an anthropoid woman. But there has to be a limit to these activities; when the stressful circumstance is over, the blood pressure and heart rate must return to normal. The parasympathetic system kicks into place at night to bring blood pressure and heart rate down, and to give the body a break from adrenergic stimulation (Fig. 1.3). So the sympathetic adrenergic system provides the response to the 'fight or flight' stimulus, and keeps us stimulated during the day after waking us up, while the

Table 1.1 Two contrasting autonomic (involuntary) systems that regulate heart and mind

	Sympathetic	Parasympathetic
Messengers	Adrenaline, noradrenaline Epinephrine, norepinephrine	Acetylcholine
Alternate names	Adrenergic	Vagal, cholinergic
Stimulated by	Anxiety, stress, danger, acute exercise	Sleep, rest, meditation, exercise training
Effects	Heart rate & BP↑	Heart rate and BP↓
Health risk or benefit	High BP; more heart attacks	BP↓; heart protection

BP = blood pressure

parasympathetic system calms the body down after the stressful event and puts us to sleep at night (Fig. 1.4).

When this balancing act is disturbed, or when the adrenergic system is over-stimulated for a period of time, then diseases of the cardiovascular system such as high blood pressure (hypertension) become more likely. In modern life, where poor diet promotes disease of the coronary arteries, adrenergic over-activity may trigger a heart attack, especially in those whose coronary arteries are already packed with cholesterol. On the other hand, in those who exercise regularly, the parasympathetic activity is enhanced, and so the chances of hypertension or a heart attack are greatly reduced.

Regulating blood volume: enter the kidney

Not all game chases ended badly for early humans, with large beasts tucking in to a hominid dinner. In fact, in order to survive, humans had to catch and eat buck, often choosing the weaker animals left behind as the herd ran away. In the Kalahari Desert of Southern Africa, members of the Khoi tribe can still outrun buck, as they have done for thousands of years. At first this seems unlikely, but humans are very well adapted to running, says Professor Tim Noakes, a world-renowned sports scientist, and author of *The Lore of Running.* Initially the buck would outrun its pursuer, but most animals have hide or fur

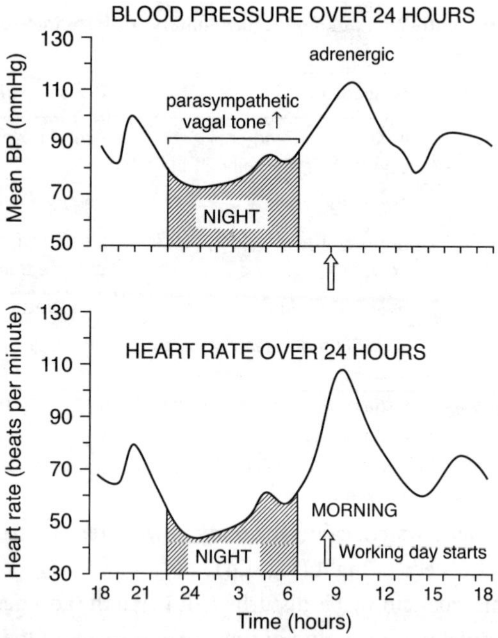

Figure 1.4 Major changes in sympathetic (adrenergic) and parasympathetic (vagal) activity—day and night. In the evening there is little stress, so that the blood pressure and heart rate are at the average, normal values. At night, both decrease, as parasympathetic vagal activity increases. But even before waking (at about 3 to 4 a.m.) both graphs start to rise, indicating the increased adrenergic activity that helps to wake us up. Highest BP and heart rates are in the early morning, at the start of the working day. The BP values shown are those of the mean BP, which, over 24 hours, was 93 mm of mercury (mmHg), corresponding to the normal value of 120/80 mmHg. © Opie.

through which it is difficult to sweat, whereas thin-skinned humans can sweat freely. Thus, after a long chase, the animals would eventually succumb to heat stroke and collapse, while the pursuing humans could keep running, staying cool by sweating, slowly gaining on their prey, and eventually catching and slaying their quarry (Fig. 1.5).

Dehydration from running

Common sense would argue that prolonged sweating during the chase would result in continued loss of water from the body, leading to

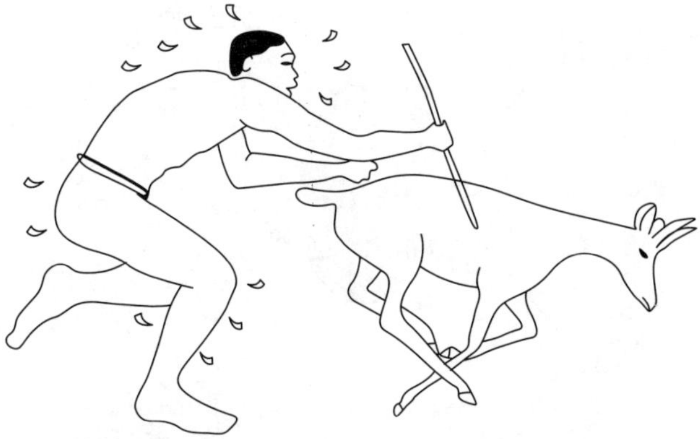

Figure 1.5 Success in the chase, achieved by chasing the buck to the point where it collapses from heat exhaustion. When running, humans can sweat far more freely than animals. But humans need to counter this acute loss of fluid by acutely decreasing the output of urine (Fig. 1.6). © Opie.

dehydration and loss of blood volume, which in turn would impair the function of the brain and heart. But this is not what happens. The key to understanding human superiority in the chase lies in the kidneys (Fig. 1.6). In response to dehydration and sodium loss, blood pressure falls. This low blood pressure stimulates the release from specialized kidney cells of a hormone called renin (derived from *renal* tissue). The effect of renin is to slow down the loss of sodium and water in the urine, and to constrict the arteries throughout the body so that the blood pressure is maintained. In this way, the kidneys saved the Khoi huntsman from dehydration, allowing him to catch the weakened and exhausted buck without himself succumbing to exhaustion and life-threatening dehydration. This is also how the kidneys step in to save the day when humans must escape danger by running fast.

Lack of salt

Our progenitors in East Africa and elsewhere did not have easily available supplies of salt. Lack of salt in the diet means that too few sodium ions reach the working units of the kidney, called the nephrons (Fig. 1.6). The result is that the kidneys developed a powerful ability to retain sodium, so that early humans could endure salt depletion.

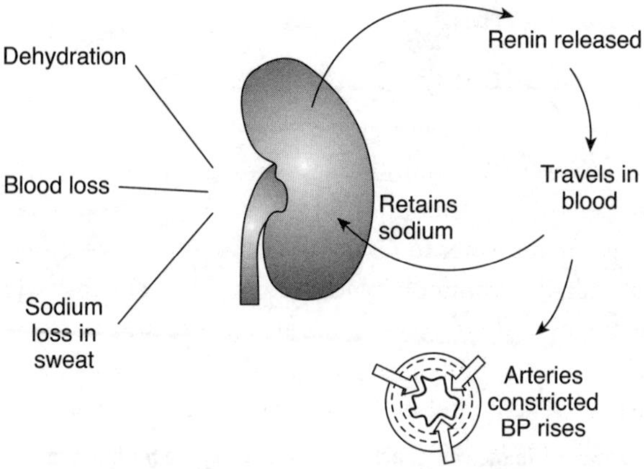

Figure 1.6 How blood loss, dehydration, or salt depletion act on the kidney. When the body suffers from loss of blood or lack of drinking water or the loss of sodium during excess sweating, the resulting low blood pressure stimulates specialized kidney cells to synthesize a hormone called renin, which is released into the bloodstream. The result is reduced loss of water and salt (sodium) from the body and better maintenance of blood pressure. Finally, too little sodium in the food, as in primitive humans often living far from a source of salt, also provokes the kidneys into holding back sodium, which is the active ingredient of salt. This primitive system saved the lives of evolving humans when salt was scarce, but now that salt in food is plentiful, the kidneys carry excess sodium back into the blood, thereby helping to promote excessively high blood pressure (hypertension). © Opie.

Effects of blood loss

This same system also protected primitive humankind after injury. When a lion or an enemy severed a limb or plunged in a spear, there would be severe blood loss. As bleeding continued, the blood pressure would drop; as in the case of salt depletion or dehydration, this would stimulate the kidney to release renin, constricting the blood vessels, and thus helping to keep the blood pressure stable in spite of the loss of blood. Low blood pressure also stimulates the sympathetic adrenergic system, which constricts the small arteries of the body, thereby keeping the blood pressure more or less constant (Fig. 1.2).

What goes wrong in disease

On the road to high blood pressure

These primitive systems, which once worked so well to enable humankind to survive tough conditions, are now accused of contributing to the problem of high blood pressure (hypertension). It is easy to see that powerful measures to retain sodium in the body, combined with the high-salt diets common in many countries, would have dire effects on the kidneys, where excess sodium is reabsorbed and passed from the urine into the blood, raising blood pressure. Furthermore, the increasing stress of modern life also promotes hypertension, as most readers will already know.

Logically, it makes sense that chronic sustained stress can drive blood pressure up in the long term, causing or precipitating hypertension. The arguments linking excess salt intake to hypertension are equally clear. These links are all real, but in fact each of the major diseases affecting heart and mind is caused by a complex array of precipitating and/or hereditary factors. Thus, quite often, excess stress stimulation is one of several factors that provoke heart attacks; the others include smoking, poor diet, obesity, hypertension, and diabetes.

Serious diseases of the heart are caused by multiple mechanisms. For example, diabetes predisposes the sufferer to kidney disease, which in turn raises blood pressure. Obesity also contributes to high blood pressure, and bad diet plays a major role in coronary artery disease and heart attacks. But the chances of developing diabetes may be lessened by switching to a healthier lifestyle, including increased exercise. This book aims to lead the reader to an understanding of—and hopefully, a commitment to—lifestyle factors that lead to the good health of the heart and mind. I suggest strongly that choice of lifestyle can promote longevity or early demise, as well as growth or stunting of the personality. The choice is yours!

Summary

The stress reaction triggered by the 'fight or flight' impulse is managed by the adrenergic or sympathetic nervous system, which increases heart rate and blood pressure, helping us to escape from dangerous situations. Conversely, the balancing system comes into play during sleep or relaxation. This is the system that protects the heart and reduces blood pressure. We can't sleep all day, but we can do exercise; paradoxically, as we shall see, this also increases the activity of the parasympathetic system, decreasing resting heart rate and blood pressure.

However, modern lifestyles promote over-activity of the sympathetic nervous system, and hamper the balancing parasympathetic system. This book will show how specific lifestyle choices can lead to the best possible functioning of heart and brain for the longest possible time. We will also touch on the prevention of cancer (beyond simply not smoking). We will be asking questions such as: which diet can best counter cholesterol deposition in the arteries? How does exercise decrease the risk of heart attacks, stroke, and diabetes? What is the Mediterranean diet, and what are its health benefits? Does drinking red wine really help? What about the low-carbohydrate (Atkins) diet? Should we worry about the glycaemic index? What about vitamins and supplements? How can memory best be retained or even improved? Can Alzheimer's disease be avoided? Does meditation alter blood pressure? We shall often be referring to the major role of the two balancing systems that operate at a subconscious level, the sympathetic and the parasympathetic systems, because the balance so often goes wrong.

Chapter 2

Long-term Health

"The heart, with the veins and arteries and the blood they contain, is to be regarded as the beginning and the author, the fountain and original of all things in the body, the primary cause of life."
William Harvey, 1628
Warden,
Merton College, Oxford

Introduction

In the previous chapter, I outlined the defence systems that the body has developed over centuries to protect itself from the environmental threats to early humankind. This chapter will develop the theme that the modern lifestyle poses special threats to the health of two vital organs: the heart and the brain. These are the major organs that need a constant supply of blood brought to them by the circulatory system—first accurately described by the Italian anatomist Vesalius in the 16th century (Fig. 2.1)—to provide oxygen and nutrients. It was William Harvey who, in 1628, established that blood actually circulated throughout the body (Fig. 2.2). This circulation is driven by the pumping action of the left side of the heart, which ejects the blood into the aorta, a large and elastic vessel through which the blood is rapidly shot on its way to the brain, kidneys, liver, stomach, intestines, and limbs.

In the limbs, the arteries narrow down until the pressure of the forward-flowing blood in the large arteries (that is, the blood pressure) drives the blood through the narrowed distal arteries, called arterioles, to reach the very small blood vessels, called capillaries. These are so thin that the oxygen easily escapes from the red cells of the blood, in which it is carried, to the tissues, which extract oxygen from the blood. The blood from which the oxygen has been unloaded looks darker and bluer than red oxygen-carrying blood. It is called

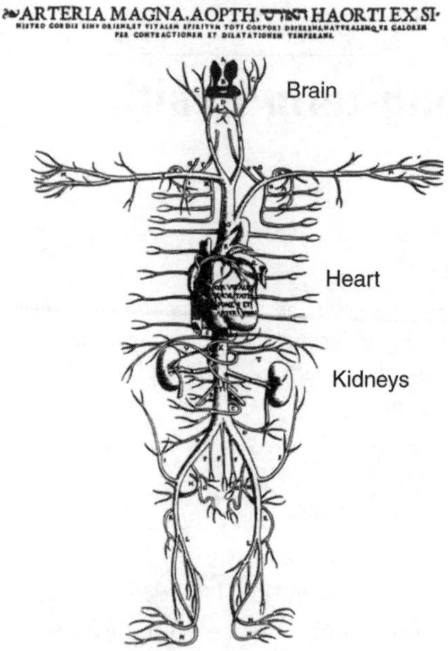

Figure 2.1 The heart at the centre of the circulation, as drawn by Vesalius (1514–1564) in his *Tabulae Anatomicae*.

venous blood, as it returns to the heart via the veins. When the arterioles are constricted or tightened, for example when exposed to icy conditions, then a higher blood pressure is needed to force the blood through to the capillaries. If that higher pressure is required all the time, then the body is experiencing the condition of hypertension, or high blood pressure.

Your lifestyle may be damaging your arteries

Our modern lifestyle promotes a disease of the arteries, called **arteriosclerosis** (arterial hardening) or **atherosclerosis** (fatty changes and hardening). Arterial damage is not spread uniformly; cholesterol-containing plaques build up in certain vulnerable sites, and each plaque has the potential to cause total arterial blockage (Fig. 2.3). Of the vital organs of the body (and every organ is vital in its own way), only two—the heart and the brain—have a blood supply that

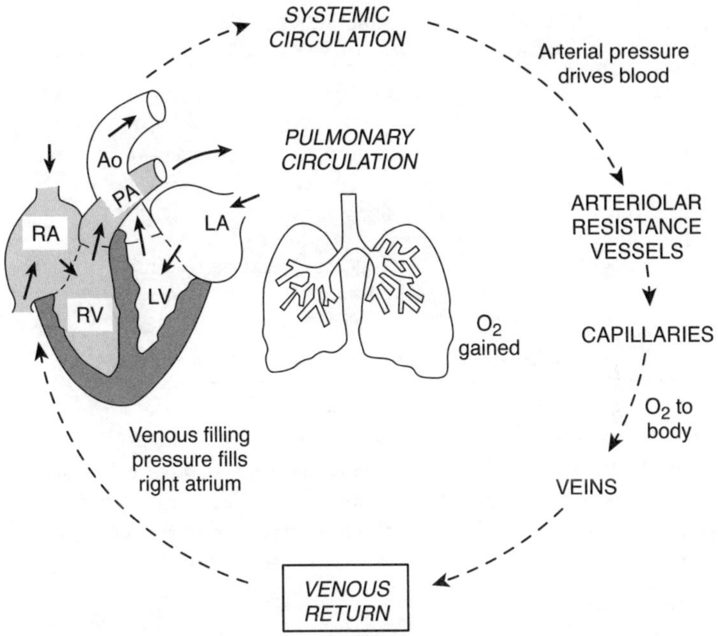

Figure 2.2 Normal circulation. In 1628, Harvey wrote: 'These are then the very elements... of the passage and circulation of blood, from the right auricle into the right ventricle; from the right ventricle by way of the lungs into the left auricle; thence to the left ventricle and aorta; whence by the arteries at large through the tissues into the veins, and by the veins back again... to the base of the heart.' Harvey used the term 'auricle', now replaced by the modern 'atrium'. In picture: RA, right atrium; RV, right ventricle; PA, pulmonary artery; LA, left atrium; LV, left ventricle; Ao, aorta; O_2, oxygen. The dotted contents of the RA, RV, and PA represent deoxygenated blood. © Opie.

can be seriously and suddenly reduced by major blockage of a large blood-delivering atherosclerotic artery, which could cause a heart attack or a stroke. You can minimize the risk of these disasters by implementing the five simple lifestyle changes discussed in Chapter 3.

Blockage of smaller arteries is less dramatic, but could potentially give rise to damage over a wider area, especially in the case of the brain; several very minor strokes can cause substantial cerebral defects, causing problems such as serious memory loss. In the heart, cumulative

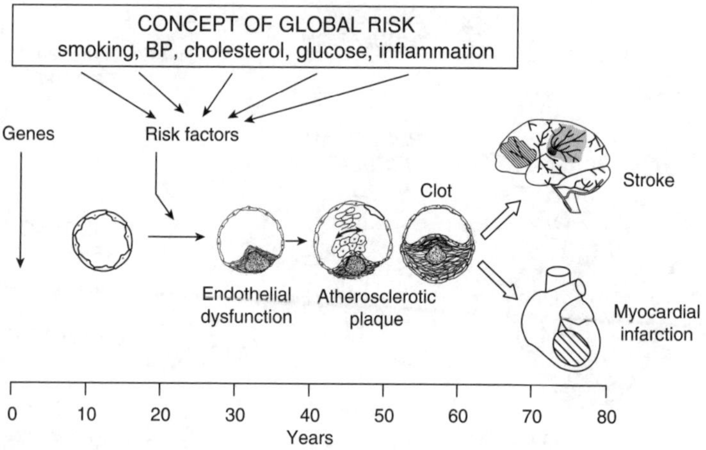

Figure 2.3 Life-long risk factors combine to cause arterial disease. Vascular disease, starting in youth, is best known to cause heart attacks, but is equally to blame for strokes. Modified from *European Heart Journal*, 2000, supplement D, by permission of Professor T Lüscher, Zurich.

small blockages can give rise to serious **heart failure**, a condition in which the heart contracts less efficiently, and fluid accumulates in the lungs and legs. Strokes and heart failure are two of the key conditions that accelerate the ageing process.

Loss of pliability of arteries

As arteries become diseased, their normal elasticity degenerates, and they eventually become rigid. This means that the pressure inside the diseased artery (or smaller arteriole) needed to deliver blood to the heart or brain must increase, in order to force the same amount of blood through the stiffened tube. In other words, blood pressure must increase, and this higher pressure further damages heart or brain cells, thereby accelerating ageing. In contrast, open and pliable arteries keep the blood flowing to the brain and heart, thus delaying ageing.

In a typical person following a Western lifestyle, the process of cholesterol-induced arterial disease starts in early adulthood. American researchers saw clear evidence of coronary artery disease in young American soldiers, aged between 20 and 25, who were killed in battle in Vietnam. Typically, these early lesions grow slowly over the years, until a cholesterol plaque becomes big enough to actually burst through the arterial wall and block the artery, causing a heart attack or stroke, usually in mid-life or later (Fig. 2.3).

How arterial damage starts

Mechanisms

We now need to consider how the arteries become damaged; and then to plan how to avoid such damage. It's widely known that cholesterol damages arteries. The technical term for such damage is atherosclerosis, a combination of 'atheroma', which means 'fatty deposit', and 'sclerosis', which means 'hardening'. Given this definition, if I said to you that the basic problem is an inflammatory process, you might find it hard to believe. After all, a well-known example of inflammation is the prick of a thorn: such a wound may become infected, and will then be surrounded by red and inflamed tissue until the inflammation subsides. Another example is acute pneumonia: the body's defence response to the pneumococcal germ produces an inflammatory response within the lung tissue. Common sense suggests that neither of these examples of inflammation remotely resembles what happens in atherosclerosis. Yet the classic article by Russell Ross in 1999 in the respected *New England Journal of Medicine*(1), explaining how coronary arteries become diseased, starts with the words: 'Atherosclerosis is an inflammatory disease.' So we have some explaining to do.

The response-to-injury hypothesis

Ross's theory is based on the *response-to-injury* hypothesis of atherosclerosis, which suggests that the process begins with an initial, cholesterol-induced injury to the inner layer of the arteries, called the endothelium (Fig. 2.4). This injury attracts white cells called monocytes—also part of the body's normal defence mechanism—from the circulating blood.

The cholesterol continues to attack the thin, delicate endothelium, making it leaky, so that both the white cells and the cholesterol molecules penetrate into the inner layers of the wall of the artery. This in turn sets up a series of characteristic lesions, each one leading to the

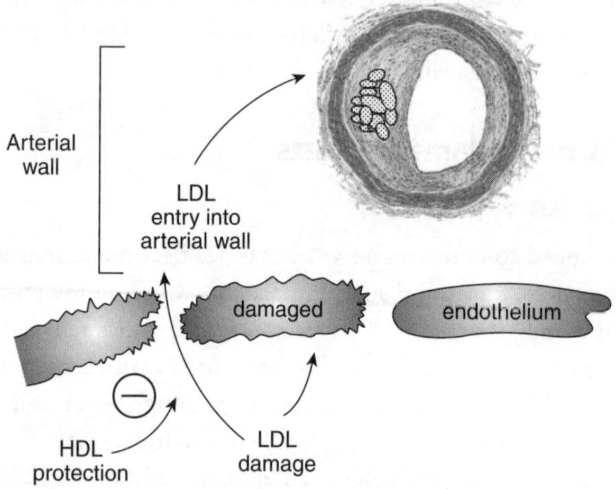

Figure 2.4 Formation of the fatty deposits (atheroma) in coronary and other arteries. The problem starts with excess circulating 'bad' cholesterol, or low-density lipoprotein (LDL), which damages the thin inner layer of the artery, the endothelium. This allows the penetration of 'bad' cholesterol through the damaged endothelium into the arterial wall. The good news is that 'good' cholesterol, or high-density lipoprotein (HDL), inhibits the entry of 'bad' cholesterol into the arterial wall.

next, each worsening step a stage in what Ross called a 'chronic inflammatory process'; not because it is an inflammation in the usual sense of the word, but because cholesterol deposits cause white cells to respond in the same way that ordinary infections cause them to respond.

Cholesterols: the bad and the good

Let us now explore the role of cholesterol in this whole disease process. Cholesterol in the blood consists of two major components. The greater part is the 'bad' low-density component—technically called LDL-cholesterol, where the LDL stands for low-density lipoproteins. These are large lipid (fat) molecules bound to circulating blood proteins, hence the term *lipoprotein.* There is so much fat in this form of cholesterol that its molecular weight is low, which explains the term 'low density'. The smaller cholesterol component consists of 'good' or high-density lipoproteins, also called HDL-cholesterol.

Almost all Westerners (and many others) have levels of 'bad' LDL that are way above the ideal. This over-supply of LDL-cholesterol damages the endothelium (the delicate inner layer of the arteries), allowing the noxious LDL-molecules to penetrate the arterial wall, becoming a foreign body within the artery (Fig. 2.4). The result is an invasion by circulating monocytes (inflammatory-type white blood cells), which penetrate the damaged endothelium and proceed to engulf the LDL-cholesterol molecules. Once these invading blood cells have gobbled up the LDL-cholesterol molecules, becoming stuffed with fat, they are called foam cells.

Plaque formation

Eventually these foam cells coalesce to form a plaque of atheroma in the arterial wall. One would imagine that this plaque would narrow the artery, but this does not happen at first. Rather, the arterial wall initially grows outwards without narrowing the artery, a process first described in 1987 by Glacov, a pathologist at the University of Chicago. However, as the plaque continues to grow, the artery eventually narrows, and blood flow is obstructed—not desirable, but hardly deadly. The disaster happens when the plaque bursts through the delicate inner layer of the artery (Fig. 2.5). Now the body's natural defence mechanisms are set in motion; in a bid to limit the damage, the ruptured area is covered by a protective layer formed by the minute blood cells called **platelets**.

Platelets normally circulate in an inactive state. When they come into contact with an exposed ruptured arterial wall, platelets become spiny in shape, and active. They promptly stick to one another, and set off signals that cause the blood to clot at the site of the burst plaque. The final result is the potentially disastrous total arterial obstruction, leading to either stroke or heart attack, depending on whether the obstructed artery is in the brain or the heart.

HDL-cholesterol: why is it 'good'?

HDL-cholesterol is good in more ways than one. First, it acts directly to protect the endothelium of the arteries from the damage caused by LDL-cholesterol (Fig. 2.4). HDL-cholesterol is a natural antioxidant that counters the LDL-induced lesions that damage the endothelium

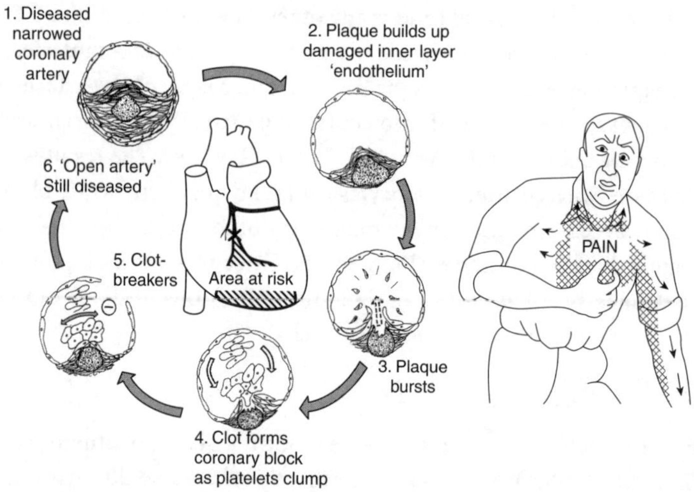

Figure 2.5 The progression from arterial atheroma to clot formation, and the therapeutic effect of clot-breaking agents. The rupture of the plaque and blockage of the coronary artery (steps 3 and 4) deprives part of the heart of its blood supply (area at risk shown in central heart), which causes an intense pressure-like chest pain, typically in the centre of the chest and spreading down the left arm, as shown on the right. Clot-breaking agents such as streptokinase or tenecteplase can restore the blood flow (step 5), as can insertion of a stent (not shown). But the artery remains diseased (step 6), so that active steps must be taken to change lifestyle and reduce cholesterol deposits to prevent a repeat heart attack. © Opie.

of the arteries and thereby promote arterial disease. Second, and not shown in Fig. 2.4, HDL can actually extract 'bad' cholesterol from the arterial wall. Third, in our laboratory experiments in Cape Town, we have linked HDL-cholesterol to the protection of heart muscle that is damaged when there is a heart attack. The protective molecular pathways concerned are now being mapped out, not only in our research, but also in the studies of Dr Joel Karliner at the University of California.

By now it is common knowledge that a low animal-fat diet decreases the blood level of LDL-cholesterol, and that there are very good drugs known as statins (Lipitor, Crestor, and the generic simvastatin, among others) that can inhibit the synthesis of 'bad' cholesterol in the liver, taking the LDL level down even further. Much less is known about ways of increasing levels of HDL-cholesterol. There are several promising medications, including long-acting niacin (vitamin B3) and various new agents not yet registered. But simple lifestyle changes, if followed, will have the same results: do more exercise, lose weight, change your diet, and take alcohol in modest amounts, as will be discussed in Chapter 3. How these increase HDL and protect against LDL is not clear, but to those living in Britain and Ireland, my tongue-in-cheek advice is to jog from pub to pub, having only one drink at each!

Heart attacks

A heart attack—technically, an acute myocardial infarction—is caused when the blood supply to the heart muscle is abruptly cut off by complete or near-complete blockage of one of the coronary arteries (Fig. 2.5). We have already learned how a person's coronary arteries may become severely damaged (Figs. 2.3 and 2.4). In the next chapter, we will discuss how to calculate the risk of that person having a heart attack in the future. Another way of looking at the problem is to ask which risk factors were present in someone who has already had a heart attack. This is the area in which the Interheart study has proven its worth.

Multiple factors conspire to cause a heart attack

In the Interheart study, Dr Salim Yusuf (formerly a Rhodes Scholar at Oxford, and now Head of Cardiology at McMaster Medical School in Canada) studied nearly 13 000 heart attack-survivors in 52 countries, with about 15 000 people (matched for age and gender) acting as controls.(2) Leaving aside the inherent risks of increasing age and male gender, Yusuf's team found that an individual's lifestyle can either protect that person from heart attack, or make it more likely to happen. The five protective factors they singled out were: not smoking, maintaining an ideal weight, regular exercise, plenty of fruit and vegetables in the diet, and modest alcohol intake.

Conversely, smoking and being overweight (the latter measured by abdominal fat) increase the chances of having a heart attack by about two to three times, as do hypertension and diabetes. Even worse were abnormal cholesterol patterns (increased 'bad' cholesterol and decreased 'good' cholesterol), which increase the likelihood of heart attack by about four times. Often several of these risk factors are present in one individual, and the effects add up—for example, obese people are more likely to have higher blood pressure and to develop diabetes.

Stress and heart attacks

This major study added a new risk factor for heart attacks, often suspected but never before clearly shown: psychological stress. Acute stress over-stimulates the adrenergic nervous system (causing the 'fight or flight' reaction), and can be linked to heart attacks as follows. First, acute stress can cause serious irregular fast beating of the heart, as shown in Fig. 6.5 in Chapter 6. Acute stress also drives up blood pressure and heart rate, thus increasing the amount of work that the heart must perform. The increased work by the heart muscle demands more oxygen in turn, and that means that more blood should flow to the heart muscle. But if the coronary arteries can't open up to carry the extra blood because of extensive coronary artery disease, the heart muscle is blood-deprived and strangulated, producing the typical pre-heart-attack chest pain (Fig. 2.5).

Furthermore, acute stress causes platelets (the small cells that clump together in a heart attack, as shown in Fig. 2.5) to stick together and block the coronary arteries. The resulting severe lack of blood flow to a large part of the heart causes the heart attack. (However, bear in mind that stress is only one of the factors promoting heart attacks, which will be discussed more fully in the next chapter.) Dr Yusuf's work teaches us that most heart attacks occur without any obvious precipitating factors, and may simply be caused by the onward creep of the arterial damage shown in Figs. 2.3, 2.4, and 2.5.

Am I having a heart attack?

However it comes about, the immediate cause of the heart attack is a blocked coronary artery, and the sooner it is opened up, the better. Ideally, this needs to happen within three hours of the onset of chest pain—typically this is a severe, constricting chest pain, like a pressure on the front of the chest, often going down the left arm, but there are many variations (Fig. 2.5). As the heart is not pumping properly, the afflicted person often suffers shortness of breath. Any sustained chest pain lasting longer than ten to fifteen minutes warrants a visit to the emergency room of the nearest hospital, where a tracing of the heart's electrical activity (an electrocardiogram, or ECG/EKG) and blood tests will rapidly diagnose or exclude a true heart attack.

The next step

Both the protective and the harmful factors documented by Dr Yusuf are covered in the next chapter. However, one of them—hypertension—merits separate consideration, as it is a powerful risk factor for stroke, which in turn is often a mercilessly disabling disease.

High blood pressure as a risk for heart attack or stroke

Hypertension, the technical term for blood pressure that is consistently higher than normal, is one of the easiest of the dread diseases to control, both because lifestyle changes can lessen the risk of hypertension, and because of the wide variety of drugs available to reduce blood pressure. Yet, according to the *Los Angeles Times* of 23 February 2010, the prestigious Institute of Medicine in the USA found that both doctors and patients often ignore the disease, even though it is 'easy to prevent, simple to diagnose and inexpensive to treat.' About one in three Americans has hypertension, which triggers about one-third of all heart attacks. And yet there are simple lifestyle measures to reduce blood pressure and prevent hypertension: a low-salt diet, stress reduction, exercise, weight loss, and increased intake of fruit and vegetables. (Diet and the heart will be analysed in Chapter 4.)

Age and hypertension

We can do something about stress, but we can't change the fact that every day, we age. Basically the arteries become less elastic over the years, so the heart must generate more and more pressure in order to drive blood through the hardened arteries. What is not always realized is that most of us now live long enough to be almost sure that we *will* become hypertensive sooner or later. The prediction is that even those who have normal blood pressure at age 55—and certainly most

Westerners—have a 90% risk of developing hypertension at some point during their lives.

Mechanisms of control of blood pressure

We know that the high blood pressure that results in a diagnosis of hypertension develops when the heart must work against increased resistance in the arterial system at the level of the smaller arteries, or arterioles (Fig. 2.6). But blood pressure varies substantially over 24 hours (Fig. 1.4), being much lower at night (when parasympathetic activity dominates), and much higher in the morning (when sympathetic activity dominates). In healthy people, the heart 'rests' at night, when blood pressure is low, then responds to early morning sympathetic stimulation, which gradually subsides during the day. So over 24 hours there is a blood pressure cycle (Fig. 1.4). And in unhealthy people? Well, the early morning 'stress' period is exactly when most heart attacks happen.

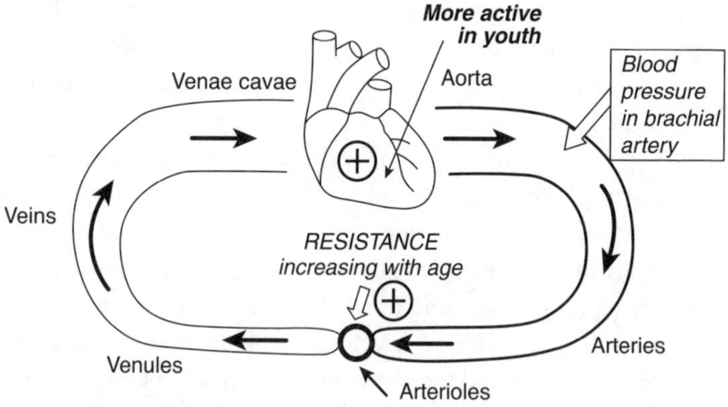

Figure 2.6 Simplified scheme of blood circulation. This shows how an increase in the resistance against which the heart works will increase the blood pressure, causing high blood pressure (hypertension). This typically occurs as the arteries harden with the passage of years. This resistance is located not in the large arteries such as the aorta, nor in the brachial arteries where the blood pressure is normally measured (Fig. 2.8), but in the smaller arteries, called arterioles, which constrict in response to adrenergic stimulation (Fig. 1.2). In younger people, increased pumping of the heart (typically in response to stress) may cause hypertension. © Opie.

'Stress' and hypertension

It is popularly believed that sustained elevation of blood pressure (that is, hypertension) is caused when repeated episodes of anxiety (and/or stress) drive up the blood pressure via sympathetic adrenergic activity. Then, in people who do not have a good balancing mechanism to bring down the blood pressure (that is, adequate activity of the parasympathetic system), or whose sympathetic system simply stays overactive, the mechanisms that enable the return of the blood pressure to normal levels don't work too well, so the blood pressure stays high. This topic will be covered in more detail in Chapter 6.

These episodes of exaggerated blood pressure rise also damage the endothelium and promote arterial damage (Fig. 2.3). But the endothelium is not just a protective layer. It is highly active, and secretes chemicals that make the arteries contract or relax, thus increasing or decreasing the blood pressure. When the endothelium is damaged, the dominant chemical messages sent to the muscle cells of the artery will promote contraction of these cells and arterial narrowing ('constriction'), thereby raising the blood pressure and damaging the endothelium even further. It's entirely possible that episodic increases in blood pressure can themselves cause or at least contribute to sustained hypertension.

Stress reduction is a complex issue, and will be dealt with in Chapter 8. Salt reduction is much simpler.

Kidneys, salt, and hypertension

The kidneys are silent workers, unlike the heart, of which we are often aware, and the brain, which guides us through our waking hours. Kidneys are also relatively silent from the disease point of view, especially when compared with the sudden and serious events that may strike the heart and the brain—heart attacks and strokes. The role of the kidneys in protecting primitive humans has already been outlined: kidneys protected our ancestors from lack of salt (sodium) in the diet by vigorously retaining sodium (Fig. 1.6). However, now that Westerners and others are eating far too much salt, often in the form of factory-made bread and butter (with added salt) or processed foods, drinks, and snacks, the retention of excessive sodium by the kidneys helps promote hypertension, and ensures that blood pressure stays up in those who already have hypertension.

Reduce salt to save lives

Indeed, if the average American were to reduce the salt in his or her diet by three grams per day (from the current average of seven to ten grams per day), the blood pressure of the entire population would drop by about as much as if every person had taken one blood-pressure-reducing tablet—and the nation would save between 10 and 24 billion dollars in annual health spending.[3] This would be one very cost-effective way for President Obama to improve the overall health of the US population, and similar arguments can be made for other Western and emerging nations. For readers who want to take this message to heart but are doubtful they can get by with less salt, be assured that after five to six weeks of salt restriction, your taste buds will have changed the messages they send to your brain. You won't miss your salt at all. In fact, the average plate of soup in a restaurant will now taste much too salty.

Why is hypertension so lethal?

Hypertension is sometimes called 'the silent killer'. Overall, the gravest danger is that hypertension will raise the pressure within the arteries supplying blood to the brain, which are surrounded by soft brain tissue. These arteries may rupture, so that blood bursts into the brain, causing a stroke (Fig. 2.7). The two major types of stroke are: (1) a brain bleed, or hypertensive stroke, caused when excessively high pressure inside the arteries bursts the arterial wall; and (2) a brain clot, when the arteries of the brain are so diseased by hypertension and cholesterol that a clot blocks the blood flow, and the brain cells die from lack of oxygen and nourishment.

Heart failure, which happens when the heart muscle becomes too weak to perform its normal work, is yet another hypertension-promoted disease. Hypertension raises the pressure against which the heart must work. To compensate, the heart muscle cells grow larger. The constant and sustained excessive work that the heart muscle must perform eventually leads to overwork fatigue and failure of the heart

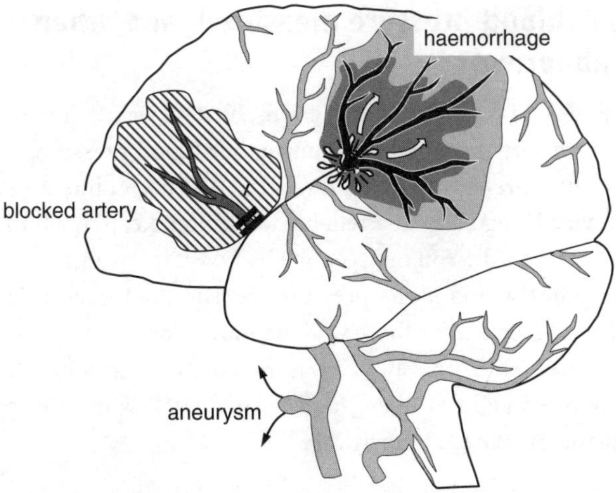

Figure 2.7 Strokes, the often incapacitating result of high blood pressure or cerebral vascular disease. Untreated hypertension (high blood pressure) can burst open one of the arteries taking blood to the brain, often at a site already damaged by LDL-cholesterol (Fig. 2.4). Arteries are blocked by LDL deposits, also shown in Fig. 2.4. Congenital aneurysms (localized dilation of the arteries taking blood to the brain) are unusual causes of strokes. Such aneurysms may burst at any age, but are (relatively) more common in young people, who otherwise have little risk of a stroke. © Opie.

cells, resulting in poor pumping function of the heart, which is potentially fatal if left untreated.

Hypertension and the kidneys

There's more. Hypertension also damages the arteries of the kidneys, eventually causing kidney function to fail. In response, the kidneys send out more of a hormone called renin (Fig. 1.6), which increases the blood pressure even further. Severe hypertension can seriously damage the kidneys, eventually requiring treatment by dialysis.

Thus it's safe to say that because arterial disease is so widespread, and because of the potent, direct effects of blood pressure on the heart, the brain, and the kidneys, hypertension is potentially the most common of all the major lethal diseases that limit health and lead to death. Fortunately, it is usually easy to treat, especially in the early stages.

How is blood pressure measured, and when is it abnormal?

If hypertension is potentially so serious, how do we nip it in the bud? We can start by repeatedly measuring our blood pressure, starting early in life, preferably in adolescence. When you buy a new car, you service it regularly at a reliable workshop, keeping all the vital details and records. You only get one body, yet few people monitor it and keep health and blood pressure records. Such precautions are especially important for those who are more likely to develop hypertension (because they have a family history of hypertension, or because they are overweight or obese) and for diabetics, who must control their blood pressure extremely carefully.

Taking blood pressure

Blood pressure varies, and there are many factors that may cause the variation: the time of day or night when the reading is taken (Fig. 1.4), the position of the person, the degree of physical and psychological relaxation, and even whether the blood pressure is taken by a doctor, at home, or by self-monitored automatic machines (Fig. 2.8). Ideally, the blood pressure should be taken several times, with the cuff on the upper arm, and when the person being tested is relaxed, sitting, and has not recently been exercising, smoking, or drinking coffee.

Often blood pressure shoots up because of the self-fulfilling fear that the doctor will find a high blood pressure. But it then falls back within the normal range when the reading is taken in more relaxed conditions—for example, by a trained nurse who knows how to lessen the emotional stress of the examination. (This temporarily abnormally high blood pressure is known as 'white coat hypertension', for obvious reasons—but it's the patient's fear rather than the doctor's coat that drives up the reading!) In clinics devoted to the detection and treatment of hypertension, patients are often encouraged to spend an hour or two sitting calmly, reading and relaxing, while their blood pressure is taken automatically by machine.

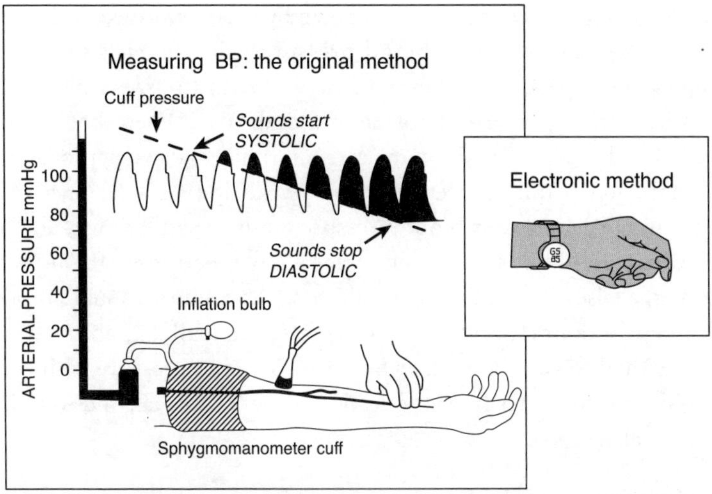

Figure 2.8 Blood pressure self-measurement: old and new technology. The standard method (left) uses a stethoscope, which conducts sounds from the cuff around the upper arm to the ears. The rubber bulb is pumped, compressing the cuff around the upper arm, until the sounds caused by the blood distending the artery with every heartbeat can be heard. This gives the top (or systolic) value. Then the pressure in the system is released, and the cuff around the arm deflates. When the sounds disappear, that is the bottom (or diastolic) value. On the right, an ultra-modern electronic 'wrist-watch' device reads out the pressure. © Opie.

Self-help

The concept of self-determination of blood pressure is becoming much more widespread, with self-test machines available in many public places, such as retail pharmacies. Also increasingly popular is self-testing at home, now that reliable, reasonably-priced home-testing machines are available. Some have a cuff that is applied above the elbow, but there is also a more modern 'wrist-watch' electronic manometer (Fig. 2.8). The wrist-watch is easiest to use, but for the reading to be correct, the wrist must be at the level of the heart—if the arm is lower than that, the blood pressure reading will be correspondingly higher.

To get reproducible results (and thereby make informed decisions about the state of one's blood pressure), the secret is to make many measurements, over several weeks, in the same physical position (sitting) and at the same time of the day. When should this be? Blood pressure climbs in the early morning, as dawn approaches; it starts to rise during sleep, to help us wake up (Fig. 1.4). Once the morning rush is over, blood pressure tends to settle down, and a reading should be taken then. After a few repetitions, the initial fear of a false high reading soon vanishes. The readings should simply be kept in a notebook or recorded electronically, enabling any individual to compare his or her average blood pressure with the ideal. But this raises further questions: what *is* normal, and what is the ideal?

What is normal blood pressure?

Years ago, hypertension was defined as a sustained blood pressure level above 160/95 units (the units being millimetres of mercury, or mmHg). Then it dropped to the current cut-off of 140/90 mmHg, with 'normal' being about 120/80 mmHg. The new ideal blood pressure is as low as about 115/75 mmHg. Values between 130/85 and 140/90 mmHg are regarded as likely to evolve into sustained hypertension. Fig. 2.8 explains how these measurements are taken, and what they mean. The top (systolic) value is potentially the most dangerous, as it usually increases with age. In contrast, the bottom (diastolic) reading spontaneously starts to drop as age progresses, so that for most people of 50 years of age or older, it is the top (systolic) blood pressure value that matters most. These values are summarized in Table 2.1.

It's evident from this table that there is a sliding scale of blood-pressure-induced damage—resting values of only about 115/75 mmHg very seldom cause heart attacks or strokes, but with each step up in blood pressure category, the danger of complications increases. Indeed, the American Joint National Council for Hypertension states that the risk of cardiovascular (heart and brain) disease rises incrementally from the ideal of 115/75 mmHg, and doubles with each increase of 20/10 mmHg.

Table 2.1 Normal and abnormal blood pressure values (in mmHg)

Blood pressure values	Blood pressure category	Action required
About 115/75	Ideal	None
About 120/80	Normal	Keep below 120/80
≤130/85 to 140/90	Pre–hypertensive	Lifestyle changes
≤130/80 plus diabetes or kidney disease	Consider as hypertensive	Treat blood pressure and underlying causative disease
≤140/90	Hypertensive	Lifestyle changes; 1–2 drugs
≤160/100	Severe hypertension	Lifestyle changes; 2–3 drugs
≤180/110	Serious hypertension	Intense decrease in blood pressure; investigate fully
≤200/120	Hypertensive crisis	Very urgent decrease in blood pressure

≤ means the blood pressure is equal to or greater than the values given

Okay, my blood pressure is normal; do I need to do anything?

To avoid future hypertension, keep your salt intake low, exercise regularly, and keep your weight down. Get into the habit of checking your blood pressure at home, and recording the results.

I already have hypertension; what now?

The same basic advice applies: keep your salt intake low, exercise regularly, and try to lose weight! And it's even more important that you get into the habit of checking your blood pressure at home and recording the results. In addition, it's vital to find a medical practitioner, specialist physician, or cardiologist who has a special interest in hypertension, and in your health. If you're on antihypertensive medications, don't neglect to take them. If you're starting off with a modest blood pressure elevation, say a systolic of 140 to 150 mmHg, your medical advisor may well aim for a systolic of about 130 mmHg.

Initial pressures of 160 mmHg or more need a slower drop, aiming to reach, say, 140 mmHg. It's important to take it slowly—over-treatment may induce symptoms of light-headedness, especially on standing up. And this is much more likely in the elderly, as their stiff arteries may fail to constrict normally on standing up.

Summary

It's essential to sustain normal blood flow to the vital organs such as the heart and brain, and the best way to do this is to keep the blood vessels supple and open. When arteries are hardened by excess cholesterol or high blood pressure, they can cause serious heart attacks or strokes. Complete blockage of one of the coronary arteries supplying blood to the heart will cause a heart attack, characterized by severe central chest pain, often going down the left arm, and shortness of breath. If you suspect that you are having a heart attack, get to the emergency room of the nearest hospital as urgently as possible, so that the faulty artery can be unblocked.

Of the many complex events that determine the health of the arteries, it is blood pressure that requires the most self-management. High blood pressure comes in all grades, from minor elevations to near-death levels. If you're interested in longevity and prolonged good health, you should learn to monitor your blood pressure yourself. The simplest precaution against inevitable age-related blood pressure rise is to cut salt right out of your diet. Other major steps are exercise and the control of body weight, which will be dealt with in the next chapter.

Chapter 3

Staying Healthy

If we knew which lifestyle habits resulted in longer and better lives, and protected from dread diseases such as heart attacks, stroke, and cancer, then we might be more motivated to modify our behaviour. Luckily, we know the answers; unluckily, we often lack the willpower to change our lifestyles. So let's first get the data—we'll assume that if it's sufficiently impressive, our new knowledge will compel us to strive for longer and better lives.

Predicting future health by a healthy lifestyle: the 'big five'

Three very large and very long studies in the USA have found five key factors that determine whether any given individual will be free of heart attack or stroke over a period of about 16 years, starting from mid-life. I have called these the 'big five' (Fig. 3.1), a term commonly used by wild game hunters in Africa. The big five (lion, leopard, buffalo, elephant, and rhinoceros) are the hardest to hunt and the most aggressive in counter-attack. Recognition of lifestyle abnormalities is the start of our hunt for health perfection, leading to strong motivation to bag the big five lifestyle-improvers.

The big five for best care of your health

The health big five of lifestyle are: non-smoking, vigorous daily exercise for at least 30 minutes, ideal weight, ideal diet, and modest alcohol. Taken together, the clear message is that when the lifestyle is perfect, there is about 80% protection from heart attacks, stroke, or cancer. And this message comes from three major studies organized by the Harvard Medical School and published in the most highly rated journals.[1–3]

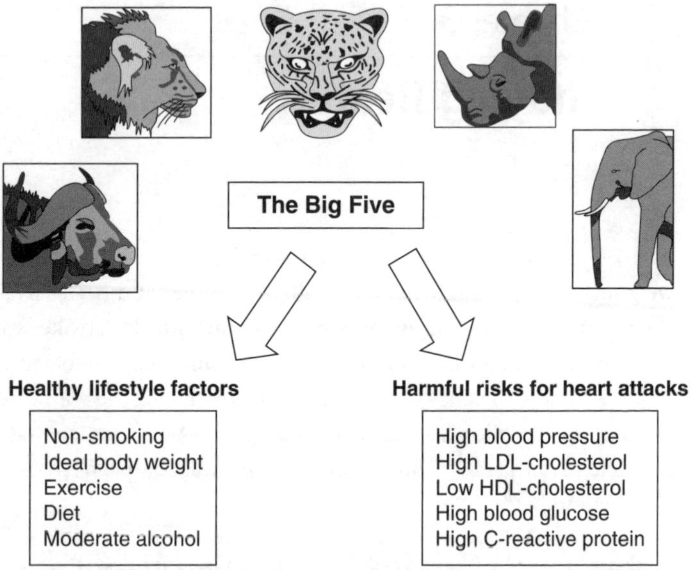

Figure 3.1 The two 'big five' groups that govern cardiovascular health. In the box on the left are the five features of the healthy lifestyle. In the box on the right are the five treatable risk factors (age and gender excluded) that need vigorous correction of any deviation from healthy blood values. The original meaning of the phrase 'big five' refers to game hunting in Africa: the 'big five' trophy animals are lion, rhinoceros, leopard, elephant, and buffalo. These were chosen according to the difficulty involved in hunting them, and not because of size. Today the phrase more often refers to game that might be seen when staying at an African game lodge, typically in South Africa, Botswana, or Kenya. Of the 'big five', the leopard is the most difficult to find—just as in humans, weight loss is the most difficult of the health 'big five' to attain! © Opie.

The studies involved two very large groups of American health professionals in which a total of 114,090 people were followed up for 16 to 18 years, giving almost two million person-years for analysis.

Note that what they analysed was how good lifestyle choices can protect us from heart attacks, stroke, and cancer. The initial study was on heart attack prevention in men, but later studies showed similar factors governing stroke prevention in both men and women, and all causes of death (including cancer) in women. Let's look at the data for women (Table 3.1), as the principles are the same for men.

Table 3.1 The lifestyle 'big five'

Lifestyle 'big five'	% of protection from deaths	Mechanism
1. Not smoking	28%	Protects arteries
2. Exercise (30 min or more per day)	17%	Slows the heart, lowers BP
3. Ideal weight	14%	Avoids toxic chemicals released from fat cells
4. Ideal diet	13%	High unsaturated fatty acids, high fruit and vegetables, low red meat
5. Modest alcohol	7%	Anti-stress; alcohol improves blood cholesterol patterns
All five	**79%**	

(Deaths from all causes, including heart attack, stroke, and cancer)

In the study, those who adhered to all five health principles proved to have almost 80% less risk of suffering heart attack or stroke than those who adhered to none of the principles. And the first three give three-quarters of the total protection (59% out of 79%). The mechanisms of these benefits are complex, as will be discussed later in this chapter.

What are the self-promoted diseases of lifestyle?

These are dread diseases promoted by the modern, sedentary, fast-food lifestyle, which started in Western countries and is now spreading to India, China, and Japan. The consequences include obesity, diabetes, and raised blood pressure, resulting in the 'modern epidemic' of heart attacks and stroke. Lifestyle changes can improve the likelihood of avoiding these major killers, and therefore of being in optimal health. However, lifestyle cannot give total protection, and certainly not from genetic factors that push up cholesterol or blood pressure or promote diabetes. Nor can lifestyle change gender or age.

Thus diseases of lifestyle may more accurately be called self-promoted diseases, because an unhealthy lifestyle increases the chances of contracting the dread diseases. To determine the chances that any given person at any given age will be the victim of a heart attack or stroke, risk factor charts must be used, and we will deal with these later in this chapter.

How feasible are these lifestyle ideals?

To adhere to all five principles may seem a tough call; and indeed, in the men's study only 4% of this educated group could adhere to all five principles and receive the maximum possible benefit. But there is good news; we can still get most of the benefit without exhausting ourselves in doing so. First, let's leave out the two aims that might be the most difficult to change in mid-life, namely achieving ideal weight and ideal diet—never fear, we will still cover these in Chapter 4. For now, let's concentrate on only the three more feasible criteria, namely non-smoking, physical exercise, and light to moderate alcohol. Combined, these can give you about two-thirds of the maximum benefit—a definite advantage over the desperate situation of those who have no beneficial components at all to their lifestyle.

What about protection of the brain?

The brain is a far more complex organ than the heart, with less well-defined criteria for damage prevention. However, we do know that stroke is a major threat to the health of the brain. In the study mentioned above, those few men and women (between two and four per cent of the sample) who managed to stick to all five principles of the optimally healthy lifestyle had a very low risk of stroke—between 70 and 80% protection. Lifestyles that protect the heart also protect the brain.

Are the American studies really relevant to non-Americans?

Because the Americans selected groups of health professionals for their studies, wasn't the focus on younger, better educated, and wealthier people? Similar studies have been carried out in Britain, where it is much easier to obtain a representative sample of the population as a whole. In Norfolk County, over 20 000 people were randomly and electronically sampled from National Health Service lists (on which nearly all British residents are registered). Trained nurses checked selected individuals to confirm the replies to questionnaires.

The study found that there were the same protective patterns of healthy living as in the American studies, and what's more, the benefits were also found in older people, and even in those who were overweight. This means that although obesity is bad, even the obese can reap the benefits of modifying the other four factors.

In the most recent study, 4886 people throughout the United Kingdom were randomly selected by computer, and followed for 20 years.(4) A health score was calculated in relation to four crucial factors characterizing poor health behaviour: smoking; fewer than three portions of fruit and vegetables per day; less than two hours of physical activity per week; and weekly alcohol intake more than 112 g (about 1–2 drinks per day) for women and 168 g (about 2–3 drinks per day) for men. The alcohol limits are similar to those found in another very large study (Fig. 3.3). Totally healthy behaviour could prolong life by 12 years compared with those who had all four self-inflicted health risks. Note that this study missed one of the big five, a really big one—weight. By missing that, their 12 year life-span difference between the healthy and unhealthy would have become, let's guess, 15 years if not more.

What about cancer?

As shown in Fig. 3.2, the greater the number of unhealthy factors, the greater the risk of cardiovascular disease (heart attacks and strokes), cancer, and deaths from all dread diseases. Out of the 'big five', the major protection against cancer is the benefit of not smoking, but the healthy diet is also important (see later in this chapter). In another study, a similar combination of non-smoking, regular exercise, moderate alcohol, and a Mediterranean-style diet (similar to the 'healthy diet' in the American studies, but with olive oil added liberally) was associated with markedly reduced 10-year mortality in elderly Europeans.(5)

Not smoking and exercise

Not smoking

Giving up smoking (or not starting in the first place) is essential: it confers just over one-third of the lifestyle benefits described above. The hazards of smoking have been well publicized by the USA Surgeon

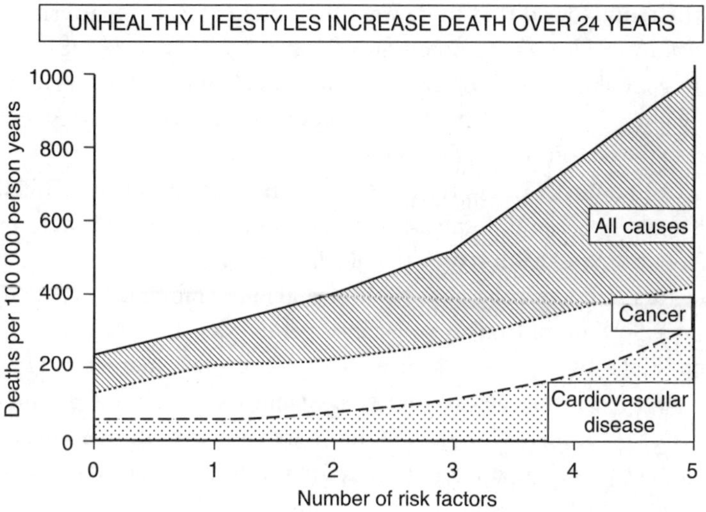

Figure 3.2 Deaths increase with the number of unhealthy lifestyle factors. A 24-year study on 77782 American women. Note the increases in the number of deaths from heart attacks and stroke (cardiovascular disease, dashed line), from cancer (dotted line), and deaths from all causes (top line). Thus, it is not only the heart that benefits from lifestyle change, but the body as a whole; there is an almost five-fold increase in all-cause deaths between those who have no abnormal lifestyle factors and those who have all five major factors. Reproduced from Dam van RM, et al. Combined impact of lifestyle factors on mortality: prospective cohort study in US women. *Br Med J*, 2008; 337:a1440 with permission from BMJ Publishing Group Ltd.[3]

General; by the government of the United Kingdom; and by authorities in many other countries where there are now regulations against smoking in public, as in India, or in shared spaces such as restaurants and pubs, as in France and South Africa. Nicotine is a potent source of damage to the endothelium, and therefore promotes arterial disease. Unfortunately, the image of smoking as being 'sexy', which was promoted for years in the USA and elsewhere, still lingers; and young women remain the group least likely to give up smoking. They need to be convinced that the long-term harm of smoking to the arteries to heart and brain, as well as the devastating and irreversible effects on the lungs, far outweigh the more immediate (and rather modest) weight-reducing effect of smoking.

Exercise

'Exercise is the elixir of life,' says Richard Verrier, from the Harvard School of Public Health. You need at least thirty minutes of moderate to vigorous exercise daily—ideally every day, but five days per week will do. How much effort should you put into it? A simple criterion: you should be sweating by the end of your exercise. The simplest way is to undertake what is called aerobic exercise, such as running or walking vigorously. How do you know if you are getting enough exercise? If you are, your resting heart rate should be about 60 beats per minute or slower. If yours is around 70 (commonly regarded as normal) you are probably under-exercised. Be warned, though: whereas you can't overdo non-smoking, exercise can be overdone. The over-trained 'athlete's heart' beats so slowly that some of the beats are dropped on the way down the conduction paths of the heart, which is also not ideal. There's a simple remedy: reduce the amount of exercise you do.

The ideal health-giving diet

Diet is a word often linked to weight loss, but the word comes from the Greek *diaita,* which really means a way of life. Thus, in its original sense, diet means the kinds of food that a person eats habitually. Currently there two separate issues: which diet best reduces weight (see Chapter 4) versus which diet gives overall optimal health and longevity.

We know that the Western diet (with its high intake of fat, sugars, and calories) damages the arterial endothelium and promotes obesity, diabetes, and heart attacks and strokes. Four validated, health-promoting diets that counter the effects of the Western diet are:

1. the **Prudent diet**, which emphasizes a pattern of high intake of vegetables, fruit, legumes, whole grains, fish, and poultry;
2. the **DASH BP-reducing diet**, which is similar in nature, but with the addition of salt restriction; it's ideal for the many people with hypertension or borderline hypertension;
3. the **Healthy Eating diet**, again similar, but using a numerical index for the seven components, each of which is given a score

ranging from 0 to 10, where 10 signifies 'optimal dietary behaviour'; and

4 the **Mediterranean diet,**[6,7] which is not that different to the others but features added olive oil and moderate alcohol; this diet has several strong points in its favour, which will be explained further in Chapter 4.

Moderate alcohol for cardioprotection?

Alcohol, the fifth protective factor (and part of the Mediterranean diet), is a two-faced friend. A little helps, but more than that harms substantially. That modest alcohol consumption can decrease overall death rates is no longer in doubt, in the light of a giant study on about a million people proving the benefits of moderate alcohol consumption (Fig. 3.3). Thus the teetotaller deprives him- or herself of the

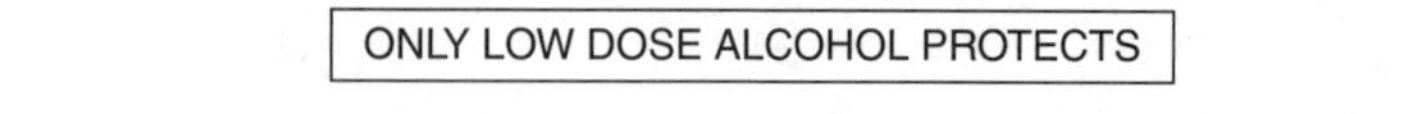

Figure 3.3 Low dose daily alcohol is protective, high dose is harmful. The peak protective effect (with a risk of about 0.85 compared with the standard) shows that a reduction of about 15% in the death rate is found in those who take only one drink per day. With 2–3 daily drinks the benefit is still there, but lessening; and at four drinks or above the benefit is lost, as the death rate rises, probably from liver damage. The J-shaped curve shows the data on 1 015 835 people gathered from a large number of different studies. (Figure based on Di Castelnuovo et al, 2006).[8]

protective cardiovascular effects of alcohol, while the heavy drinker is laid low by the direct toxic effects of excess alcohol on the liver and other organs and by increased car accidents and violence. Also of note is that it seems as if very little alcohol is needed to achieve this protection—especially in women, who have (on the whole) a lower liver capacity to break down alcohol; so that up to 2–3 drinks per day is protective in men, but women need only 1–2 drinks for similar protection.

Proof that modest alcohol intake truly protects the heart

Modest alcohol intake may just reflect a relaxed lifestyle. Proof that alcohol really protects the heart comes from studying a group of people who have an uncommon genetic deficiency in the liver mechanism that breaks down the alcohol in the blood.(9) There are two main consequences of this condition: first, the rate of breakdown of alcohol by the liver is much slower, with higher than normal levels of alcohol in the blood, as we might expect. But second, this group suffers far fewer heart attacks than is considered normal. Alcohol stimulates the liver's production of protective, 'good' (high-density lipoprotein, or HDL) cholesterol. Thus modest alcohol intake protects those at risk of stroke or heart attacks.(10)

Red wine versus other alcoholic drinks

The 'red wine hypothesis' states that red wine has benefits extending beyond its alcohol content.(11)

Red wine and experimental heart attacks

Supporting the red wine hypothesis, strong data come from dogs with experimentally narrowed (stenosed) coronary arteries, which is a model of human coronary artery disease.(12) In these dogs, administration of an expensive French Bordeaux red wine, Chateau Neuf-du Pape (as a dose of 4 ml/kg, given into the stomach), allowed the blood to flow more freely in the coronary arteries because of a strong inhibitory effect on blood clot formation. Deep red grape juice (natural, purple juice, without additives) had the same effect, but in a higher dose of 10 ml/kg. These dog doses would translate into human daily doses of about 300 ml of red wine and 750 ml of purple grape juice daily, both within easy reach of human intake (750 ml equals one standard bottle of wine). Similar experiments have never been done on humans. Interestingly, white wine had only very modest effects on these dogs. Why?

Resveratrol is often held to be one of the major protective components of red wine. Many experiments on rodent hearts have shown undoubted protection against induced heart attacks, but the corresponding doses for human protection would be far too high to be practical. But basing their comments on current experiments on rodents, some researchers go so far as to say that resveratrol is the forerunner of a new group of drugs (the 'caloric restriction mimetics'). These act in a manner similar to that of decreased calorie intake, thereby opposing the effects of overeating, and prolonging lifespan. At present there is still a vast difference between treating rodents and treating humans; but in the future, newer chemical compounds developed from resveratrol will probably be discovered or created, with the prospect of halting the current epidemic of obesity sweeping the Western world.

Human data on red wine

An ingenious experiment separated the effects of alcohol from the effects of the non-alcoholic contents of red wine. Humans with coronary disease were treated with red wine from which the alcohol had been removed (technical term: 'de-alcoholized'), and protective effects were reported.[13] A daily dose of 250 ml (one-third of the size of a standard wine bottle) of de-alcoholized Greek red wine decreased stiffness of the aorta, the key blood vessel that conducts blood from the heart to all the major organs of the body. The indirect implication is that drinking that amount of red wine will increase blood flow to the heart and brain. Overall, the amounts of resveratrol and related compounds found in some red wines, such as good pinot noirs, are likely to be just enough to help to counter the vascular events that predispose to heart attacks.[11]

Does the French Paradox support the red wine hypothesis?

The catchy term 'the French Paradox' was invented and promoted by the wine-loving French (much as the concept of 'extra virgin' olive oil was invented and promoted by the Italians!). In the popular mind, the French Paradox is the inexplicable (but, it must be said, still hypothetical) capacity of the French to eat all the fatty items (such as *foie gras* and cheese) that they want, provided that these fatty foods are washed down with much red wine. As attractive as this concept seems, the hypothesis that drinking any wine, whether white or red, can undo the sins of gluttony and excess fat consumption remains to be proven.

A stringent French look at the existing data by Professor Ducimetere appeared in a recent issue of the journal *Dialogues in Cardiovascular Medicine*, which was devoted to articles on the French Paradox[14]. This review shows that where one lives (the geographic position on the north-south latitude) might be more important than belonging to any particular country, even France. Thus it is chiefly the southern, Mediterranean part of France that has the low cardiovascular death rate. Indeed, the protective effect of living in Mediterranean Barcelona, in Spain, is as strong as that of living in Mediterranean Toulouse.

This view emphasizes that France is a country divided by diet, with different cardiovascular event rates from top to bottom, and specific cities no different from those in other countries at similar latitudes. Thus, the real paradox is why the French Paradox continues to exist as a concept, when it should be replaced by a less mystifying view—namely, 'the more Mediterranean, the better'.

What are my chances of having a heart attack or stroke?

Now we move from lifestyle, which is how you live your life, to what aspects of the health of the heart and brain can be measured to give your specific risk factors for heart attacks and stroke. The degree to which you adhere to the ideal lifestyle should give a good indication of how you should fare. But suppose you have inherited high blood cholesterol, or blood pressure that stays high despite the beneficial lifestyle—then you need to know what your specific chance of a future heart attack or stroke might be.

Knowing your risk factors allows you to work out the chances of being free from heart attacks or stroke for the next five years.

Unfortunately, similar calculations for cancer prediction are not yet available. Risk factors for heart attacks or strokes give a fairly accurate glimpse into your future health. For example, high blood pressure increases the risk of having a stroke; the higher the pressure, the greater the chances of a stroke. However, though lifestyle can easily be self-assessed, evaluating the risk factors is a little more complex. But with a little effort, risk factors can also be self-determined; you don't need to go to a medical doctor to find out your risk of a potentially fatal heart disease.

The risk factor hypothesis

Whether heart attacks and strokes occur depends chiefly on the amount of cholesterol in the arteries that take blood to the heart or brain, and on the blood pressure, both of which confer a certain risk. Of the major risk factors, two can't be changed—age and gender. Age is easy to understand: as you grow older, your arteries become weaker and incur more damage. Why gender matters may seem directly related to protective female hormones, but even long after menopause, women seem to have hearts about ten years younger than those of men of the same age. Of all the other risk factors, there are five that can be changed: blood cholesterol, blood pressure, smoking, blood sugar (glucose), and a newly-added fifth risk factor—a measure of the degree of 'inflammation' in the body. Let's leave aside the complex issue of inflammation for the time being, and see what we can do about the other four factors.

Risk factor studies

There have been several major studies that may guide us in our quest to predict the risk of future heart attacks or strokes. The Framingham study was the first, and is still the best. In the 1960s, a group of epidemiologists turned their attention to a small New England village. They examined almost all the inhabitants, and undertook follow-up studies many years later. Then, for the first time, they could link initial cholesterol levels to later heart attacks, for example. Another abnormality noted at the initial examination was high blood pressure, which could be linked to later heart attacks and strokes. This study is the most famous and most used in predicting who is at risk of heart attacks and strokes, and in deciding on preventative treatment such as lowering cholesterol or blood pressure. The data from the study have been fed into risk factor charts. The charts I like to recommend for lay persons are those evolved by the Gaziano brothers, at Harvard Medical School.[15]

The Gaziano Harvard risk factor charts

These do not require any blood samples to be checked for cholesterol levels, thus simplifying self-diagnosis (see Fig. 3.4 for the Harvard

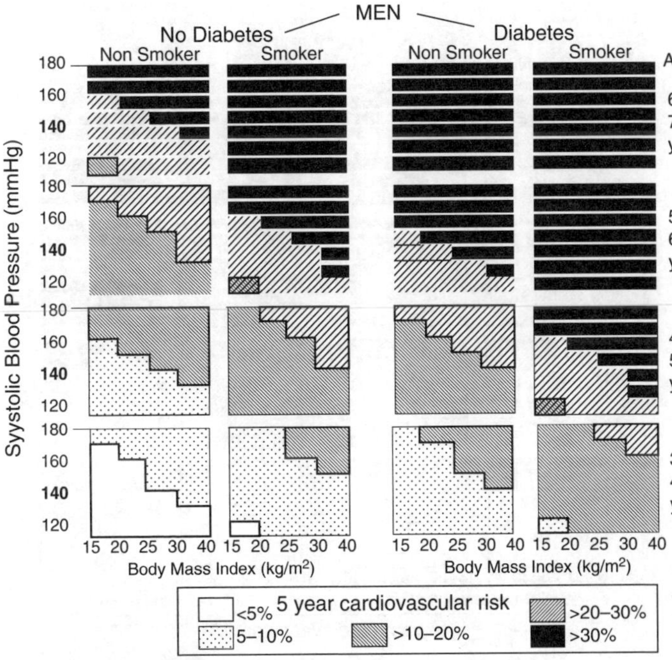

Figure 3.4 Harvard risk factor chart for men, predicting cardiovascular risk (heart attacks and stroke) for the next 5 years. Major risks that are arbitrarily divided are diabetes or no diabetes, and smoking or non-smoking. The graded effects are those of blood pressure, body mass index (BMI), and age (up to 74, no data for higher age). Diabetes, smoking, and increasing age make the worst risk combination for any given BMI and blood pressure. Women have a similar pattern but with lower risk for any given combination of risk factors. Courtesy of Thomas Gaziano MD, Brigham and Women's Hospital, Boston. Modified from Gaziano TA, et al., with permission from Elsevier[15].

Chart for men and Fig. 3.5 for women). Surprisingly, blood cholesterol does not feature at all, and that distinguishes these charts from all the others that determine cardiovascular risk. The Gaziano charts replace the measured blood cholesterol by body mass index (BMI), which relates body weight to height, correlating surprisingly well with the level of blood cholesterol (Fig. 3.6). Measurement of blood glucose is replaced by a history of the prior presence or absence of diabetes.

The lowest risk is for those at values of BMI at or a little below the 'normal' of 25, with a top ('systolic') blood pressure below 120 mmHg,

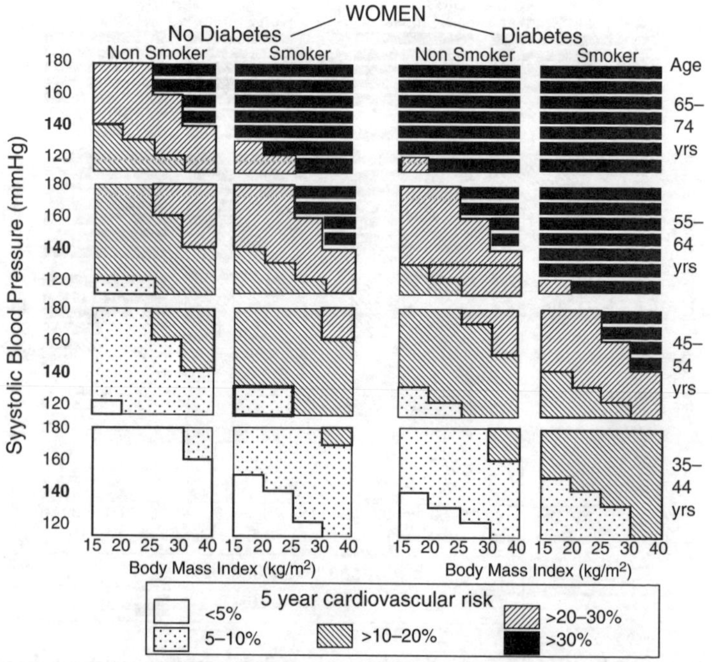

Figure 3.5 Harvard risk factor chart for women, predicting cardiovascular risk (heart attacks and stroke) for the next 5 years. Women have a similar pattern to men (see Fig. 3.4), but with lower risk for any given combination of risk factors. For women the approximation is: subtract 10 mmHg off the male blood pressure value, thereby moving two blocks down on the BP scale and lessening the overall risk. Courtesy of Thomas Gaziano MD, Brigham and Women's Hospital, Boston. Modified from Gaziano TA, et al., with permission from Elsevier.[15]

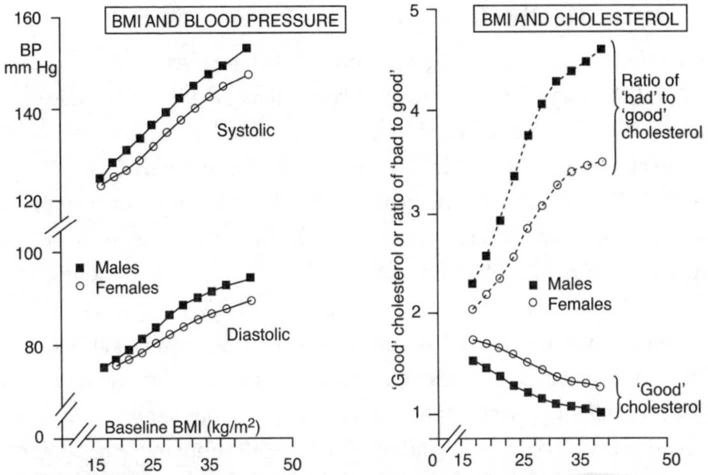

Figure 3.6 How body weight, measured as the body mass index (BMI), affects blood pressure and cholesterol. These data come from a very large and long study on nearly one million people. Because taller people weigh more, the weight is related to height by the body mass index, which is calculated as weight in kg divided by height squared in metres, wt/ht^2). Note the consistent increase in blood pressure values with weight, with men having higher values than women. Also note that the ratio of 'bad' to'good' cholesterol increases with BMI. Women have higher values of 'good' cholesterol, which in part explains their greater longevity. Modified from Prospective Studies Collaboration, Body-mass index and cause-specific mortality in 900 000 adults: collaborative analyses of 57 prospective studies, *Lancet* 2009; 373: 1083, with permission from Elsevier.

non-smoking and non-diabetic, and, of course, being a younger woman rather than an older man. (The charts confirm that women fare better than men, for any given age.) One of the factors giving women better protection is their genetically higher values of 'good' (high-density lipoprotein, or HDL) protective cholesterol. Once such non-invasive estimation of risk has been completed, then any person at higher than expected risk for age and gender can go ahead to explore the risk more exactly by blood measurements of 'bad' (low-density lipoprotein, or LDL) cholesterol, 'good' HDL cholesterol, and fasting blood glucose. For such refinements, it is best to work with a family doctor or cardiologist.

How to use the Gaziano charts

First decide—are you diabetic or not? If you are overweight and have a family history of diabetes, regard yourself as a diabetic for these purposes. Then get your blood pressure measured, which can easily be done at a pharmacy or clinic (or even at home if you have the equipment). Calculate your body mass index by dividing your weight in kilograms by the square of your height in metres (for Americans, measure your weight in pounds and height in feet and inches, and then find the American Cancer Society and BMI on Google). The Gaziano charts give the combined risk for heart attacks and stroke (that is, the total cardiovascular risk) over the next five years. Below 5% is excellent, 5–10% for a non-smoker probably requires weight or blood pressure reduction, and over 10% needs more investigation; for example, a full lipogram, giving all the cholesterol components and the fasting blood sugar (and probably also the index of inflammation, or C-reactive protein), and a visit to a family physician. A risk of over 20% means there is a one in five chance of you having a major cardiovascular disease in the next five years, which is serious enough to require urgent attention and vigorous attempts to reduce the unacceptably high risk, both by lifestyle changes and by medication.

The fight against fat

One of the five key criteria for optimal health is a body mass index (BMI) of 25 or below (Fig. 3.6). Excess body fat is bad news for the heart, especially when located in the waist. Consistent studies show that fat around the middle—abdominal fat—is closely linked to increased heart disease and diabetes. In fact, abdominal obesity causes a twofold increase in the risk for heart attacks. Are you in this category? To find out, all you need is a simple tape measure. In America, the guideline is that waist measurements exceeding 102 cm (40 inches) in men and 88 cm (35 inches) in women indicate dangerously disease-prone waistlines. European and (especially) Asian limits are much lower.

To understand the relation between abdominal fat and disease, we must dip into current research. This shows that fat is not only cosmetically undesirable, but that fat tissue produces a variety of hormones, each of which is capable of adverse effects. For example, release of these hormones from fat tissue into the blood can trigger a series of chemical changes that eventually produce even more fat. In brief, fat produces fat.

Body fat and heart disease

There are at least two major links between abdominal obesity and heart disease. First, obesity predisposes you to hypertension (Fig. 3.6), one of the major dangers for both heart and brain. Second, current research shows a directly linked sequence of events that (in some predisposed subjects) eventually leads from obesity to diabetes. And diabetes spells a very poor health prognosis. For example, a middle-aged person with diabetes but no history of heart disease has the same high risk of a future heart attack as a non-diabetic who has already had one heart attack. Walking down any Western supermarket aisle and eyeing the waistlines on show will tell you how common abdominal obesity is.

There is a potentially dangerous condition that helps to explain the links between obesity and subsequent diabetes: the metabolic syndrome.

Five key features of the metabolic syndrome (Fig. 3.7)

These are abdominal obesity (defined as above), high or only modestly elevated blood pressure, low blood HDL ('good') cholesterol, increased blood triglyceride (that is, the actual fat in the blood), and a modest elevation of blood sugar, short of diabetic levels. Having any three of these five symptoms qualifies for the diagnosis of metabolic syndrome, but some experts say that the most important factor is abdominal obesity, a view that I support. And even if your total blood cholesterol seems normal, the 'good' can be too low and the 'bad' too high. The bottom line is that the metabolic syndrome not only makes you pre-diabetic, but also predisposes you to heart attack.

Occurrences of the metabolic syndrome are increasing at an alarming rate throughout the world, but especially in sedentary populations of industrialized societies such as the USA and Western Europe, as well as those in India and China. Weight reduction (tackled in the next chapter) is crucial to the management of both obese hypertensives and the metabolic syndrome, besides being a cornerstone of the successful control of diabetes.

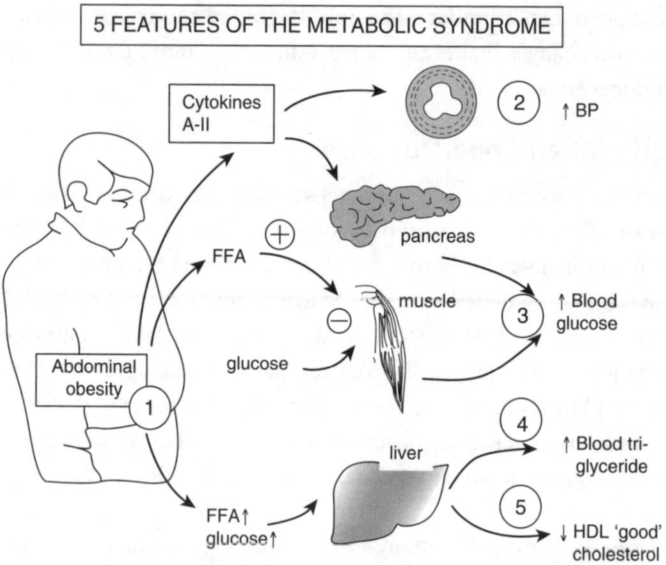

Figure 3.7 The metabolic syndrome: a risk for future diabetes and heart attacks. The five basic features are as follows: abdominal obesity; raised blood pressure (BP); increased plasma glucose above the normal limits; increased blood triglyceride (a measure of the fat globules in the blood); and decreased 'good' HDL cholesterol. Any three or more of these clinch the diagnosis. According to the International Diabetic Federation, and supported by the Cape Town hypothesis, the crucial abnormality is number 1. The excess of abdominal fat cells releases excess free fatty acids (FFA) into the bloodstream to explain abnormalities 3 to 5. The increased BP is in part explained by the increased release from the abdominal fat cells of vasoconstrictor inflammatory cytokines, and the hormone called angiotensin-II (A-II), both of which raise blood pressure. The basic remedy: lose that abdominal fat. © Opie.

'Fat women, thin women suffer for science'

As a junior doctor (working in the Toronto General Hospital in Canada at the time), I wondered whether fat people were fat because they did not break down fat stores sufficiently rapidly during the no-food period, or whether they were fat because they made too much fat just after a carbohydrate meal. With my colleague, Paul Walfish, we decided to test the former possibility. We selected a group of ultra-fat women and another control group of ultra-thin women. Both groups had agreed to exercise vigorously.

The headline in the Toronto Star read: 'Fat women, thin women suffer for science'. We found that exercise in fat women evoked different changes in blood free fatty acids (FFA in Fig. 3.7) from exercise in thin women. These fatty acids are used by muscle during exercise; they must not be confused with cholesterol, which is not a fatty acid, but rather a totally different type of fat. The greater rise in blood fatty acids in thin women meant that the fat stores of the thin women were more mobile and could break down quicker. Thus, the fat women had a double disadvantage. They generally exercised less than their thin counterparts, meaning they had fewer periods in which fat stores could be broken down to blood fatty acids. But even when exercising, their fat stores would be released into the blood more slowly than those of thin women. Thus the fat women, though they had more fat stores, were also less capable of breaking fat down and getting rid of it, so fat loss was more difficult for them. This finding, some readers would say, is proof that life is not fair.

Ways by which fat makes fat

Abdominal fat is now classed as an active organ that makes many hormones. For example, *adiponectin* is a hormone that promotes the metabolic breakdown of glucose in other organs such as muscle and liver. However, in the metabolic syndrome the levels of adiponectin are decreased, making an increase in the blood glucose level more likely. Abdominal fat also produces many hormones, probably more than any other organ in the body. *Resistin* is a hormone that inhibits the effects of insulin on muscle, so that more insulin is required to clear the blood of the rise in glucose after a meal. In this way, insulin is made less effective, which puts the pancreas under strain because it must produce more insulin. This resistin-caused combination of high blood insulin and high blood sugar is the state of *insulin resistance*, which is a forerunner of overt diabetes. It's probable that the very fat women we studied in Toronto were in an advanced state of insulin resistance.

Abdominal fat also stirs up inflammation in the arteries (see next section), rendering them more likely to be damaged by high blood cholesterol levels or by high blood pressure. Thus, excess abdominal fat also causes increased risk of heart disease and hypertension.

The new risk factor: 'tissue inflammation'

Here's the background: the body reacts to foreign material (such as an invading bacterial germ) by mounting a healthy counter-attack, in the form of a protective inflammatory response. How this happens is that the circulating blood changes in two distinctive ways: white blood cells increase, and the blood levels of protective proteins produced by white blood cells also increase. One of these proteins is called C-reactive protein, and it is singled out because it can be measured easily. The white cells (or leucocytes) that normally counter-attack bacterial infections are usually the large ones (called monocytes) that develop into macrophages (from macro = large, and phage = eater, for obvious reasons).

Adipose tissue forms nasty chemicals for export

This process is all well and good. But current research suggests a very unexpected and intriguing link between fat cells in fat tissue (technically called *adipocytes*) and disease in other organs, because of this process. In a nutshell, it looks as though abdominal fat can poison all the vital organs. Abdominal fat liberates free fatty acids into the blood, as we learned all those years ago in Toronto. These launch a reverse attack back onto the adipocytes, where the fatty acids stimulate the formation of the more modified white blood cells.

The next steps are more complex. An example of the normal function of white cells is to respond to a skin infection by clustering around the site of a bacterial infection and pouring out defensive proteins that attack and destroy the infectious bacteria. Now, let us go back to the modified white cells produced by adipose tissue. Even though there is no infection to combat, these adipose tissue cells liberate similar proteins, which now start to attack blood vessels throughout the body, as already shown for the heart in Fig. 2.4. Such white cell induced attacks occur not only in the heart, but in skeletal muscles, the pancreas, the liver, and other organs—probably including the brain (Fig. 3.8). Because of the important role that normal white cells play in the defence against bacterial inflammation, this abnormal mechanism is also called

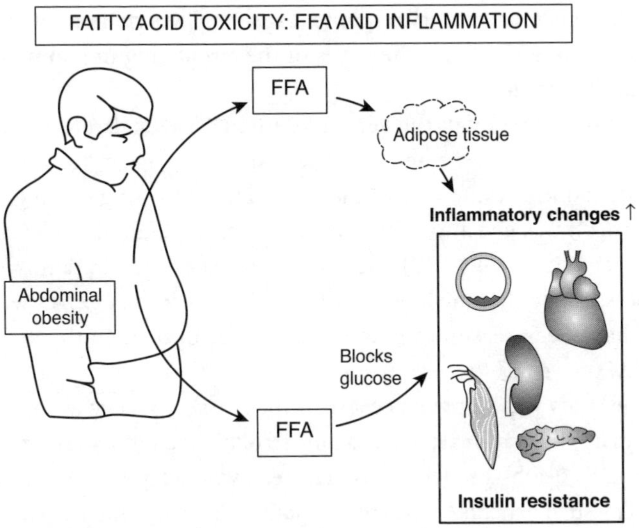

Figure 3.8 New research: obesity promotes tissue inflammation. Free fatty acids (FFA) released from abdominal fat into the bloodstream again reach adipose (fat) tissue, to activate immune cells in the fat tissue. These cells release chemicals (technical name: cytokines) that further promote inflammatory damage in the arteries, heart, skeletal muscle, kidney, and pancreas.(15) These changes combine with the block of glucose metabolism induced directly by the high blood FFA levels (Fig. 3.7) to interfere with the protective effects of insulin. The end result is that the action of insulin is impaired (insulin resistance). Because insulin normally lowers the blood glucose, obesity readily leads to diabetes. © Opie.

an inflammatory response, which of course is very confusing. In common parlance, this is known as poisoning the vital organs, which is much less confusing.

How can we treat inflammatory damage to arteries?

This abnormal inflammatory response does not yield to standard anti-inflammatories such as aspirin or non-steroidal anti-inflammatories (NSAIDS). Rather, we need to find an agent that decreases blood cholesterol (and therefore cholesterol in the coronary arteries). Cholesterol-induced damage to the coronary arteries acts like a foreign body and invokes the inflammatory response (Fig. 2.4). Thus cholesterol reduction should also reduce the levels of the circulating inflammatory-induced proteins.

In a major study in the very influential *New England Journal of Medicine* in 2008,[(17)] a new cholesterol-lowering agent, rosuvastatin (trade name Crestor, one of the cholesterol-lowering statin group of drugs), was given to people with excessively high blood levels of C-reactive protein (CRP)—the blood marker of the inflammatory process. Note that the blood cholesterol levels in themselves would not have been reason to prescribe this type of drug in the normal course of events.

The study was stopped because of the marked beneficial effects of the drug, in that heart attacks and stroke were cut by about half. Crucially, deaths also fell.[(16)] Therefore, it would have been unethical to deny such benefits to the control patients who had not received the statin drug. These remarkable results also strongly suggest that a simple blood test for CRP could help in deciding whether or not to treat a borderline cholesterol value using a statin. For this reason, many cardiologists and other specialists now include this test in any assessment of the cardiovascular risk of their patients.

Lifestyle change becomes real

The ideal course of action for any given person is dedicated adherence to as many of the five lifestyle measures as is possible, but this is a vast challenge for most of us. Sometimes it is really difficult to persuade even educated patients that lifestyle modifications are necessary, or that they could be effective. The three lifestyle measures that are most likely to be followed, in order, are:

1. the most popular one, namely modest alcohol—or for teetotallers (and less popular), purple grape juice;
2. non-smoking; and
3. daily vigorous exercise.

The reward of virtue

Even after the assault of a heart attack, human beings are reluctant to modify their behaviour. This is demonstrated by the results of a study of three critical lifestyle changes, namely improving diet, increasing exercise, and giving up smoking.[18] Indians had the highest rate (at about 90%) of diet change and of cessation of smoking, whereas Australians did best (60%) at increasing exercise levels. South Africans resisted change most stubbornly, as only 25% undertook exercise, and only 40% stopped smoking or changed their diet. Overall, those who adhered most to the three changes did best, with fewest repeat heart attacks. On the other hand, we know from current studies in the USA that there have been three key protective events there: more active therapy in treating high blood pressure; more active therapy in treating high cholesterol; and smoking has declined. The result is that in the USA, the rate of occurrence of acute heart attacks is steadily going down.[19]

Perfect values

But we're not there yet; in fact, even the perfection we're aiming for may not be as optimal as we think. The values of cholesterol and blood pressure that we now see as acceptable may still be above the absolute ideal. If we look at isolated, non-developed, non-smoking populations, we see even lower figures that are considered normal. For example, a study done on a small tribe of indigenous people in Brazil, with a physically active, non-sedentary lifestyle, found that the average total cholesterol of the tribe is only about 3.1 mmol/L (120 mg/dL), and the average top (systolic) blood pressure is about 100 mmHg.[20]

Have I missed the boat?

If I am 65 or 70 years old, what is the point of my undertaking lifestyle modifications such as starting to exercise or losing weight? Certainly, stopping smoking at any age is beneficial from the cardiac point of view, and would stop the progression of chronic lung disease. But do I really need lifestyle changes at my age?

One of the major purposes of lifestyle modification (especially in the presence of obesity or the metabolic syndrome) is to avoid the onset of diabetes, which brings with it a whole new complexity to life. In the Diabetes Prevention Programme, reported in the *Lancet* in 2009, those who began lifestyle intervention after the age of 65 had greater protection from developing new diabetes than those who started while under the age of 45.[21] Thus, better late than never.

Summary

There are five major lifestyle features that protect from heart disease and stroke (leaving out age and gender, which cannot be changed). The lifestyle 'big five' are: not smoking; avoiding obesity; moderate to vigorous daily exercise; ideal diet; and modest alcohol consumption.

The major warnings of impending disease that can be measured and therapeutically corrected are another 'big five': higher than normal blood pressure; increased blood glucose; two blood cholesterol components, namely the 'bad' low-density lipoprotein (LDL) and the 'good' high-density lipoprotein (HDL); and fifthly, the recent arrival: ultrasensitive C-reactive protein (usCRP), a marker of the tissue inflammatory response. Several of these abnormalities are grouped together and known as the metabolic syndrome, for which a warning sign is increased abdominal girth. This increasingly common pre-diabetic condition also yields to lifestyle changes.

Chapter 4

Diets for Modern Living

"The peoples of the Mediterranean began to emerge from barbarism when they learnt to cultivate the olive and the vine."
Thucydides, 5th Century BCE.

"UNESCO considers adding the Mediterranean diet to intangible World Heritage List"
Newspaper report, August 27, 2010.

The major purpose of 'going on a diet' is usually either to lose weight or for medical reasons such as threatening cholesterol problems, incipient diabetes, or hypertension, to achieve better protection of the heart and brain. But what about simply feeling better and living longer? Remember the 'big five' of the Good Long Life: non-smoking, exercise, ideal weight, ideal diet, and moderate alcohol. As already discussed in Chapter 3, exercise is pretty simple—a daily average of 30 minutes or more of moderate to strenuous exercise. The reasons for not smoking are obvious, and moderate alcohol consumption is within easy reach for those who are not alcoholics or teetotallers. This leaves the far more complex issues of how to control body weight and how to find the ideal diet, which are the topics covered in this chapter.

Of course, the perfect answer to the worldwide increase in obesity would be prevention. To start with, over-feeding in early childhood must be avoided. Indulgent parents and grandparents are often to blame for wanting a 'healthy, chubby baby' rather than instilling life-long patterns of restrained food intake. Start prevention even earlier say modern nutritionists—weight gain by the pregnant mother sets the scene for an overweight baby.

For the person who is already overweight, which is the best diet? And what is a diet in any case? The word originates from the Greek *diaita*, meaning 'a way of life'. Thus the original meaning in ancient

Greece referred to the pattern of food habitually eaten over a long time, which was part of a pattern of life that included exercise. The second (more modern) meaning implies restriction of the type and amount of food, most usually to reduce weight.

When I praise the Mediterranean diet, I mean a traditional pattern of eating that goes back to ancient Greece, and is now known to lead to long-term health benefits. The ideal would be if the Mediterranean dietary pattern became the modern norm. By contrast, most weight-reducing diets are short-term calorie-restricted efforts to overcome long-standing obesity.

Principles of weight loss

Principle number one: combine diet with exercise

All diets work best with increased exercise. I emphasize to patients that the combination to strive for is 'fewer calories in' and 'more calories out', and the latter is achieved only by exercise. Which type of exercise is best? It should be sustained and involve repetitive movement, such as running on a treadmill, vigorous swimming, cycling, or fast walking. For best results, we should exercise daily for at least half an hour, but preferably an hour (some experts recommend an exercise-free day per week).

Principle number two: persist, persist, persist

Starting any chosen diet may be easy, but adherence is not. Time and again studies show that when diets are tackled with enthusiasm, there is temporary weight loss. But after a few months, about two-thirds of those who start don't continue and lapse. This was shown in a study at Tufts University, Massachusetts, which tracked four groups of dieters following different regimes including the Atkins and the Weight Watchers diet. After one year, adherence to the allocated diet was the only common factor in those who lost weight.

Adherence is greatly improved by group classes and enthusiastic dieticians. In a large Harvard-based study done over two years, the single factor that linked to sustained weight loss was not the type of diet followed, but the regularity with which participants attended fortnightly counselling sessions. Not unexpectedly, paying participants also promotes adherence, as shown in one study from Stanford, California.

When workers have lunch as a main meal together in a staff cafeteria where the diet can be carefully monitored and strongly encouraged, there can be very high adherence even over a two-year period, as seen in a recent major Israeli study.[1] In other words, group pressure helps adherence. The lone individual, told by his or her medical practitioner or sports trainer or beauty confidant to lose weight, will need determination of steel.

If so many fail on different diets, who actually succeeds?

In my view, the crucial issue with any diet is *the very strong and sustained willpower to follow it.* The motto is: 'Strong Minds Overcome Fat'. Besides the intellectual knowledge of what and how to eat, there must be a dedicated emotional driving force. In the definitive study on successful long-term weight losers, quoted in the scientific journal *Nature* in March 2004, three factors that distinguished nearly 3000 successful dieters from unsuccessful participants were: first, they were on calorie-restricted diets; second, they closely monitored their weight and food consumption; and third, they exercised for more than one hour a day. It seems that these successful dieters must have had a strong and sustained determination to succeed.

Which diet has the best long-term data?

Here we must switch focus from the concept of diet to that of dietary food pattern. The modern Western food pattern is not a healthy one. It promotes obesity, raises blood pressure and cholesterol levels, and results in more heart attacks and diabetes. Conversely, the traditional Mediterranean dietary pattern is beneficial on all these scores—though without reducing weight unless there is added calorie restriction. Overall, the following rule holds: body weight is a balance between calories in and calories out, whatever the diet.

Let's first look at the traditional Mediterranean dietary pattern, its composition and its benefits. Then we'll turn to the low-carbohydrate Atkins-type diet and its potential for faster weight loss.[1]

The protective Mediterranean pattern

Seafood from early evolution to the industrial age

When our human predecessors 'split' from apes, those who lived near the sea or large rivers where fish were abundant and accessible had the evolutionary advantage. This is the 'aquatic ape hypothesis'. The fish oils would have been helpful in the development of a large brain, thereby giving an advantage in the struggle for existence. Today, the usual diet in industrial countries contains much less fish oil than the diet of a century ago, which in turn had much less fish oil than the diet of early hunter-gatherers. There is strong evidence to show that several of the so-called diseases of civilization can be countered by increasing dietary fish oils, as found in the Mediterranean diet.

Who discovered the Mediterranean diet?

The turning point was the landmark Seven Countries Study. By chance, a great American pioneer epidemiologist, Ancel Keys, had a holiday home near Naples. He noticed that longevity was more common and that the diet there was different from that in middle-class America. He then undertook a rigorous worldwide study of seven different countries, and found the lowest incidence of heart attacks in those living on the Mediterranean islands of Corfu and Crete, leading to the concept that the traditional Mediterranean dietary pattern is the gold standard.

Is the evidence strong?

Since then, a series of studies has proven that the Mediterranean dietary pattern (Fig. 4.1) has excellent long-term epidemiological evidence in its favour. Furthermore, the more Mediterranean the better as judged by the nine points of the diet that constitute the ideal (Table 4.1). What additional hard evidence would be required to prove that the Mediterranean diet actually improves cardiovascular health? The European Society of Cardiology recognizes that the risks of a heart attack are lower in Mediterranean countries than in the rest of Europe. However, it is one thing to provide evidence that populations who eat a more Mediterranean diet live longer and have fewer heart attacks, fewer strokes, and possibly less cancer, but it is much

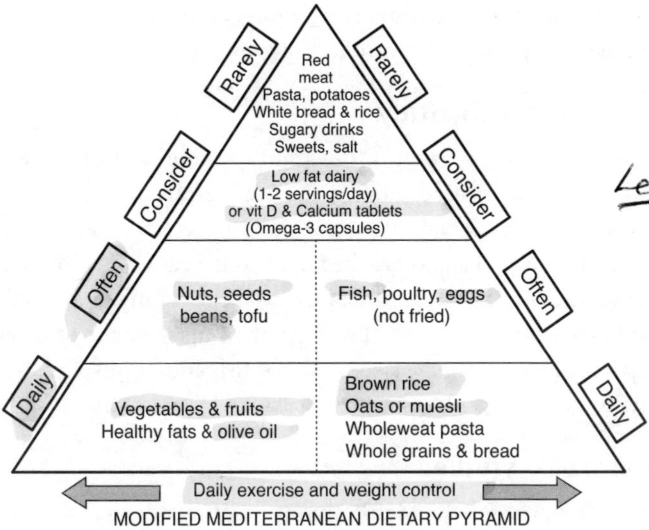

Figure 4.1 The Mediterranean dietary pyramid. This figure presents the traditional Mediterranean diet, rich in vegetables, fruit, healthy oils such as olive oil, and whole grains, with fish and poultry instead of meat. Modified from Supplement 2 to Shai, et al. 2008[(1)] by addition of omega-3 capsules, which should be given to all who have had heart attacks or are at high risk of heart attack.

Table 4.1 Traditional nine-point Mediterranean diet

High intake foods	**Low intake foods**	**Points gained**
fresh vegetables	Meat, meat products†	1 + 1
fruits and nuts	Dairy products (fatty)†	1 + 1
legumes		1
cereals		1
fish		1
olive oil†		1
modest alcohol		1

†(giving a high monounsaturated to saturated fatty acid intake)

Trichopoulou A, et al. *N Engl J Med* 2003; 348: 2599.

more difficult to prove convincingly direct cause-and-effect, which needs well-designed and controlled long-term comparative studies.

A crucial French study

In a group of French patients, all within six months of a heart attack and living in the south of France, the Mediterranean diet did better than the standard post-heart attack diet. It protected patients from repeat heart attacks and strokes over four years of follow-up.[2] Overall, there was increased dietary intake of a range of beneficial blood fats and dietary fibre. Probably the single change of greatest significance was the increased intake of fish and of olive oil, which contains linolenic acid, an omega-3 fatty acid (Table 4.2).

Supporting studies

Further support for the Mediterranean diet relates to a large post-heart-attack study conducted in Italy. After experiencing heart attacks, patients were advised to increase their intake of fish, fruit, raw and cooked vegetables, and olive oil. Those who adhered most strictly to the Mediterranean dietary pattern reduced their risk of death by half.[3]

Table 4.2 Types of fats in food

1. Unsaturated fats
• Monounsaturated fats, e.g. oleic acid in olive oil (one unsaturated bond)
• Polyunsaturated fats, e.g. omega-3 fats in fish oils (several unsaturated bonds)
• Omega fatty acids have an unsaturated bond 3 carbons from the end:
◦ omega-3, e.g. linolenic acid; ECA or DHA
◦ omega-6, e.g. linoleic acid (18 carbons)
◦ omega-9, e.g. oleic acid (18 carbons)
• Transfats, e.g. trans oleic acid (Fig. 4.8)
2. Saturated fat, e.g. palmitic acid (16 carbons)
For oleic, linoleic, linolenic, and trans fatty acids, see Figs. 4.6 and 4.8.

ECA, eicosapentaenoic acid, polyunsaturated 20-carbon fatty acid (Fig. 4.7); DHA, docosahexaenoic acid, polyunsaturated 22-carbon fatty acid.

But is it really so surprising that the results of studies in Mediterranean countries such as the south of France and Italy support the Mediterranean dietary pattern? Are there not many obvious differences in lifestyle to that found in the USA and Northern Europe, which might amplify the benefits of the Mediterranean diet? Another study, this time conducted in America (Chapter 3, Ref. 7), showed that those following a Mediterranean diet pattern had reduced all-cause death rates, including deaths from heart attacks and strokes. The percentage reduction in all-cause mortality was 20 per cent in both men and women. The reduction in cancer, though found, is probably only small, as discussed in Chapter 3.

Of course, these studies only show the association of the Mediterranean diet with better health, *without proving cause and effect.* For example, those Americans who chose this diet might have been better educated and more able to afford such a diet. For strict cause-and-effect proof, we must rely on the French and Italian studies on patients with prior heart attacks.[2,3]

How important is olive oil?

Liberal amounts of olive oil are used in the Mediterranean countries, and 30–40 grams daily of extra virgin olive oil was part of the Mediterranean diet in the Israeli study.[1] This means that the Mediterranean diet is really a high-fat one, although the fat is largely unsaturated. Olive oil is mostly oleic acid, an unsaturated fatty acid (18:1) with the bond in position 9 (omega-9), but not in the optimally protective omega-3 position (Table 4.2). High-quality virgin olive oil has added cardio-protective components—in technical terms, these give it antioxidant and anti-inflammatory properties.

Good and bad cholesterol

When the Mediterranean diet includes either added virgin olive oil or nuts, there are beneficial decreases in blood glucose and blood pressure, as well as increased 'good' cholesterol and modestly decreased 'bad' cholesterol.[4] The reason we say cholesterol has 'good' virtues and 'bad' vices is that the good cholesterol keeps bad cholesterol out of the arteries (Fig. 2.4). Thus the Mediterranean diet is one of several dietary measures to increase good cholesterol, technically called high-density lipoprotein (HDL) cholesterol.

A diet supplemented with olive oil also reduces the index of tissue inflammation, C-reactive protein (CRP). Another major benefit of olive oil when used for cooking is that it mostly replaces other cooking oils such as sunflower seed oil. The latter lacks the crucial omega-3 bond that has been proved to offer protection (Table 4.3).

How virgin is extra virgin?

Only the Italians could have come up with the phrase 'extra virgin'. Extra virgin olive oil is freshly cold-pressed from olives of superior quality. Thereafter it is kept in the dark at a low temperature to avoid changes induced by sunlight and heat. It has the very best taste, colour,

Table 4.3 Three criteria to prove benefits of polyunsaturated omega-3 fatty acids (omega-3-FA)

First, is there convincing laboratory data? Yes, omega-3-FAs inhibit currents involved in potentially fatal fast irregular heartbeats (ventricular arrhythmias); in animals fed high omega-3-FA diet, less damage to the heart is seen in model heart attacks.
Second, are there long-term population studies? Yes, many (intake of oily fish offers protection against heart attacks in the Japanese and Greenland Inuits, for example). Blood triglycerides are lowered. In an 18-year follow-up study, men with highest blood levels of the 22-carbon chain omega-3 fatty acid were 38% less likely to develop serious irregularity of the heart beats (atrial fibrillation).†
Third, are there large double-blind trials of therapy? Yes, in a large Italian study of those who had a recent heart attack (the GISSI study), omega-3-FA capsules (1000 mg/day) improved outcomes by 10–15% and decreased sudden cardiac death. A similar study on heart failure patients gave a more modest 8% benefit. In a third study in Japan (JELIS), omega-3 capsules were given to persons with high blood cholesterol, reducing coronary events by 19%; this trial was not blind. A fourth trial showed that low doses (376mg/day) gave no protection from repeat heart attacks.* The established total dose is 1000mg/day, the total of EPA and DHA, not total fish oils.

†Virtanen JK, et al. Serum long-chain n-3 polyunsaturated fatty acids and risk of hospital diagnosis of atrial fibrillation in men. Circulation 2009; 120: 2315–21.
*Kromhout D, et al. New Engl J Med 2010; August 29; online.
For reviews, see Lavie CJ, et al. J Am Coll Cardiol 2009; 54: 585–94 for positive endorsement and Jenkins DJA, et al. CMAJ 2009; 180: 633 give restrained views.

and aroma—and costs more. It is one of the few oils that can be added to food without first undergoing any preparation or chemical processing. It can be eaten immediately, and retains the natural flavours, vitamins, minerals, antioxidants, and other healthy products of the ripe olive fruit. This extra virgin oil should be kept in the dark to avoid changes induced by sunlight. In a recent study from the *British Journal of Nutrition*, virgin oil did not change the level of 'bad' LDL-cholesterol, but made it more resistant to oxidation, essential before cholesterol is taken up into the coronary and other arteries. Unfortunately, 'extra virgin' oil was not studied.

Olive oil decreases blood pressure

The more Mediterranean the diet, the greater the blood pressure reduction, as was found in a European study. The oleic acid in olive oil is the specific component that opens the arteries of the body and thus reduces blood pressure.(5)

Why nuts?

Fresh, unsalted, unbaked nuts are part of the Mediterranean diet. To achieve a one per cent reduction in 'bad' LDL-cholesterol, the following daily doses are needed: 4 g walnuts, or 11 g pecans, or 4 g peanuts, or 4 g pistachios. Almonds in large amounts, about 75 g per day, increase 'good' HDL-cholesterol and decrease 'bad' LDL-cholesterol. Adding nuts to the Mediterranean diet, as was done in the Israeli study, has a better chance of reducing the risk of new diabetes than does increasing the virgin olive oil content of the diet.(6)

Why doesn't the Mediterranean diet present the same problems as a high-carbohydrate diet?

After all, it is a high-carbohydrate diet. However, olive oil delays gastric emptying, especially when combined with vinegar, which is standard in Mediterranean countries. The absorption of carbohydrate foods is delayed, so that after the meal the blood sugar (glucose) rises more slowly and reaches a lower peak. The result is a lowered glycaemic index, as well as modestly decreased total cholesterol and triglycerides in the blood. Fasting glucose levels also drop. Indeed, the more Mediterranean the diet, the lower the incidence of new diabetes.(7)

Which fish should be eaten?

There is universal agreement that the best choices are the oily fish, which contain protective omega-3 fatty acids; for example, tuna, salmon, swordfish, mackerel, trout, and sardines. Two populations that traditionally eat loads of oily fish, the Inuits and the Japanese, both have low incidences of heart attack.

Ecological issues

Now that eating fish has become trendy and there are sushi bars on every corner, the latest problem is that fish are vanishing from the oceans as a result of over-fishing. In addition, no-one knows the effect of global warming on the fish supply. One solution is to establish more fish farms, as in Japan and elsewhere. Long term, however, as the fish message takes root and fish becomes more and more expensive, omega-3 capsules (pure EDA and DHA) will become an alternative.

Freshwater fish

Sea-dwelling fish are not the only fish to offer these benefits. As tests from Lake Superior show, fish from a cold freshwater environment—including lake herring, lake trout, salmon, and whitefish—are as high in omega-3 fatty acids as saltwater fish. Nile perch from Lake Victoria are also high in omega-3 fatty acids. Unfortunately, keeping these large lakes clean and full of healthy fish means an environmental battle with chemical companies and humans who contaminate the water.

A caution

We often hear about the dangers of mercury in fish. In reality, mercury is lowest in wild salmon, which for all practical purposes is mercury-free (Table 4.4). Farmed salmon should be totally free of mercury, but careless fish farmers sometimes give these fish mercury-contaminated food. Therefore, I support the advice of the American Heart Association: no salmon or other oily fish for pregnant mothers or growing children, because of the possible harmful effects on the brain of even traces of mercury. Instead, pregnant mothers should take omega-3 capsules.

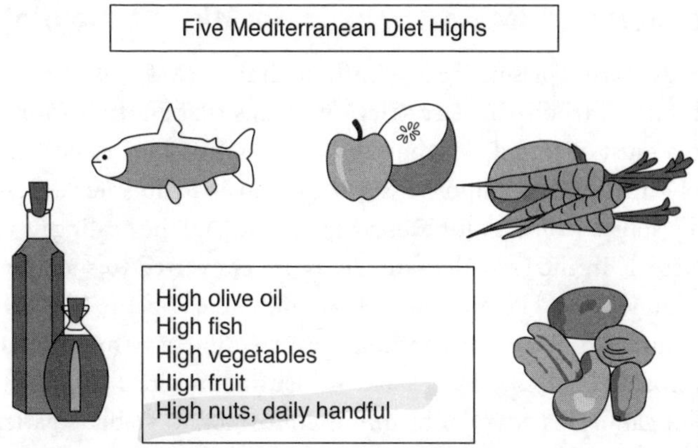

Figure 4.2 The Mediterranean diet Five-H mnemonic. To remember the dietary pyramid shown in Fig. 4.1 is no easy matter. When faced with a choice of food in a supermarket or at home or in a restaurant, this simple mnemonic will help.

Conclusion on Mediterranean diet

I like to summarize the beneficial Mediterranean dietary pattern using a five-H mnemonic: High olive oil, High fish, High fruit, High vegetables, and a Handful of nuts every day (Fig. 4.2). However, to lose weight, calories *must* be restricted.

Table 4.4 Average mercury concentration in various fish and shellfish

Fish/Shellfish	Concentration (parts per million)
Swordfish	0.97
Albacore tuna	0.35
American lobster	0.31
Chunk light tuna	0.12
Cod	0.11
Pollock	0.06
Catfish	0.05
Salmon	0.01

Source: Northeast States for Coordinated Air Use Management; Food and Drug Administration.

The modified low-carbohydrate Atkins-type diet

The basic principles of the low-carbohydrate diet (Fig. 4.3) are two-fold. First, carbohydrate restriction means that another source of energy must be found, which must be fat, as protein does not readily supply energy. Thus adipose tissue breaks down to liberate fatty acids, a good source of energy for exercising muscle, and the beating heart in particular. In the liver the fatty acids are converted to short-chain compounds called ketone bodies that inhibit the appetite (Fig. 4.4).

Secondly, the Atkins diet abruptly decreases the carbohydrate intake that normally elicits the release of insulin, and insulin promotes weight gain. This effect of insulin is confirmed in diabetic patients, who gain weight once they are put onto insulin injections. However, the increased intake of saturated fats and cholesterol in Atkins-type diets defies the common understanding of a 'healthy' diet.

Probably the best study of the Atkins-type diet was the Israeli study in which the 'low carbs' concept was modified for cafeteria use where dietary guidelines could be strictly implemented (Fig. 4.5). Besides 'low carbs', participants were strongly encouraged to use vegetarian sources of fat and protein and to avoid harmful transfats (which will be explained later in this chapter and in Fig. 4.8). This study is well worth analysing carefully. It is limited only by the rather small number of subjects in each group (just over 100), by the subjects being mostly male, and by the very unusual circumstances, in that all participants worked in an Israeli research centre, where their daily lunches (the main meal of the day) were tightly organized in a food-controlled cafeteria.

Participants were allocated the modified Atkins-type diet, the Mediterranean diet (also modified by calorie restriction), or the American Heart Association low-fat diet. In the modified Atkins diet most of the energy was provided by fat at 41%, versus protein at 32% and carbohydrate at 28%. Corresponding values for the Mediterranean diet were 32% fat, 25% protein, and 45% carbohydrate. Enthusiastic and careful dieticians and kitchen workers guided participants by labelling each item of food 'free to consume' or 'consume in moderation', as well as giving the carbohydrate, fat, and calorie content. Of the three diets, the modified Atkins-type diet was not calorie-restricted,

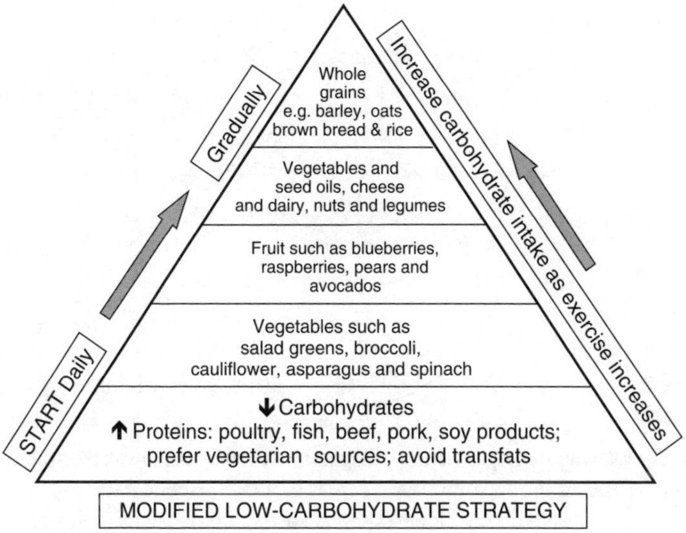

Figure 4.3 The modified low-carbohydrate high-fat dietary pyramid. Low-carbohydrates, starting with 20 g per day and then working up while maintaining weight loss. The life-long plan is 45–100 g of carbohydrate per day. Note that seed oils such as olive oil are an important part of the pyramid, as are nuts and whole grains. Participants in the Israeli study were advised to eat vegetarian sources of fat and protein and to avoid transfat. Fat was the major source of energy at 41%, and carbohydrate the least at 28%. When compared with the Mediterranean diet pyramid in Fig. 4.1, the major differences are the prominent position given to red meat at the bottom of this pyramid versus its position at the top (i.e. most sparing use) of the Mediterranean pyramid. Whole grains at the bottom of the Mediterranean pyramid become the top and least used in the low-carbohydrate pyramid. Figure based on information in Shai et al. 2008.[1]

Disclaimer: Although every effort has been made to depict the diets actually used in the study by Shai et al., this figure is not intended to replace reference to, nor the use of, the original Atkins diet, for which the following book should be consulted: *Dr Atkins New Diet Revolution*, R Atkins, Vermillion, 1992. Note the concepts of the Carbohydrate Ladder (p.171) and the Critical Carbohydrate Level (p.195).

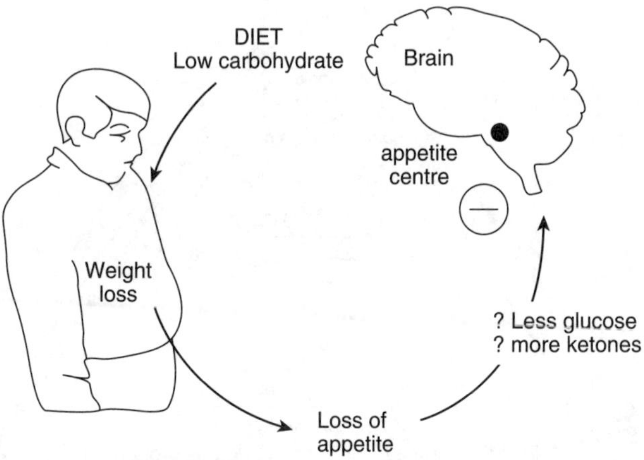

Figure 4.4 Proposed hypothetical mechanisms whereby the low-carbohydrate diet suppresses the appetite. The theory is that low carbohydrates mean that body fats are broken down. This increases blood levels of ketones, which inhibit the appetite centres in the brain. © Opie.

whereas the other two were. In practice each group consumed about 1300 kcal per day, because of the appetite-restricting effects of the modified Atkins-type diet. All participants also increased their levels of exercise.

The major endpoint of the study, weight loss at 24 months, was almost identical for the calorie-restricted Mediterranean diet and the modified Atkins-type diet, although the latter took effect more quickly, with participants reaching peak weight loss of about 6.5 kg after only four months (Fig. 4.5). Both diets saw a levelling off at about 5 kg of weight loss overall, an improvement on the low-fat diet, where weight loss levelled off at about 3.5 kg. Paradoxically, the blood fat changes were unexpectedly beneficial in the modified Atkins-type diet, and the worst in the low-fat diet. The major change seen in blood lipids was a greater increase in 'good' HDL-cholesterol in the case of the modified Atkins-type diet than in the low-fat diet.

Despite the increased dietary carbohydrate in the Mediterranean diet, it was almost as effective as the modified Atkins diet in decreasing blood triglycerides and increasing HDL. This effect of a high-carbohydrate diet is contrary to expectations. To decrease blood

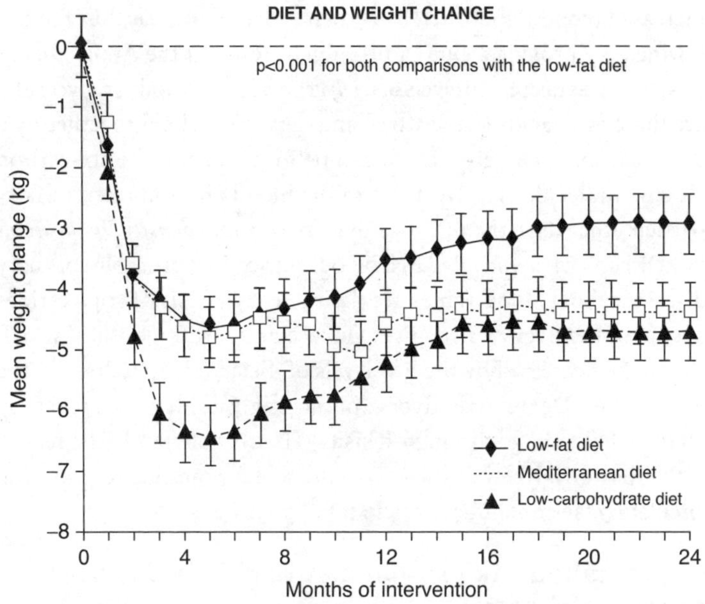

Figure 4.5 Two competing diets give the same weight change after two years. The low-carbohydrate diet was a modified Atkins diet, and the Mediterranean diet was traditional but calorie restricted. Both gave better weight loss results than a standard low-fat diet. All groups lost weight, but the reductions were greater in the Atkins and the Mediterranean groups ($p<0.001$ for interaction between diet group and time). Reproduced from Shai I, et al. N Engl J Med 2008; 359: 229–41, with permission of the *New England Journal of Medicine*.

triglyceride and to increase HDL, the Mediterranean diet must act differently in some way from the Atkins diet. It is possible that the high oleic acid content of olive oil inhibits the enzyme that produces circulating triglyceride from other, larger, circulating fat molecules, and this fall in triglyceride will indirectly increase HDL-cholesterol.

Some complex explanations—*skip unless you feel compelled to read.* The possible explanations for these lipid changes are not clear, and involve technical material that only the avid reader need follow. The intervening steps between decreased dietary carbohydrate and increased blood ('good') HDL-cholesterol are not clear, but the following may provide a clue. A prominent result of the Atkins diet in this study was decreased levels of *triglycerides* in the blood. Triglycerides are three fatty acids (hence 'tri-' and 'glyceride') held together by a three-carbon fragment, which can be formed from the six-carbon glucose molecule. Triglycerides in the blood are contained in fatty particles that have the technical names *very low-density lipoproteins* (VLDL) and *chylomicrons.* High blood triglycerides promote coronary disease, so low blood values are desirable. Synthesis of triglycerides occurs in the liver and requires glucose and insulin, both of which should be decreased by the low levels of dietary carbohydrate in the Atkins diet. Decreased adverse blood triglyceride is mirrored by increased blood ('good') high-density (HDL) cholesterol. The reason is that both triglyceride and HDL compete for binding to a specific circulating fat-containing protein (apolipoprotein).

Is a modified Atkins-type diet beneficial in cases of severe obesity?

There are no long-term studies. One comparison of the Atkins-type low-carbohydrate diet with the low-fat diet showed a short-term benefit of the Atkins diet versus a standard low-fat diet with less than 30 per cent of the calories from fat.[8] The Atkins diet was modified (somewhat like the Israeli study) to encourage a high intake of fruit and vegetables high in fibre. Those on the Atkins diet were not calorie-restricted, but spontaneously reduced calorie intake. I speculate that by breaking down fat, the Atkins diet increases short-chain breakdown products (ketones) in the blood, which may inhibit the appetite centre (Fig. 4.4). In absolute terms, in this study (as in others on obesity) the maximal weight reduction from the mean starting level of 130 kg was modest—just below 6 kg for the Atkins diet, and below 2 kg for the low-fat diet. The modified Atkins diet improved the response to insulin, and was therefore anti-diabetic.

Does the Atkins-type diet have any effect on the incidence of heart attacks?

Proper randomized long-term studies to answer this question would extend over several years and would involve a large number of people, randomly allocated to years of strict adherence to the Atkins or another rival diet. Such studies would be practically impossible. But some good guesses can be made from the findings of the large Nurses' Health study in the USA, which took place over 20 years.(9) In those who ate the low-carbohydrate diet plus high vegetable fat and protein, the incidence of heart attacks was modestly reduced.

Studies such as these—which observe, but do not attempt to alter what happens in any given group of people—are called *observational*, and provide no direct proof of cause and effect. Thus long-term, carefully monitored studies of the modified Atkins diet are now needed, specifically in comparison with established cardioprotective diets such as the Mediterranean diet and DASH diets (for more on the DASH diet for hypertension, see below).

What about the failure of carbohydrate restriction in the Harvard study?

This is one of the largest and longest studies to come to the simple, scientifically sound conclusion that calorie restriction reduced weight, irrespective of whether the diet was low-fat and high-carbohydrate or high-fat and low-carbohydrate, as in the Atkins diet.(10) However, 64% of the low-carbohydrate group were female American college graduates, who were (presumably) well-informed, and who started off with a diet already low in carbohydrate (44% of total calories). There was no change in carbohydrate intake during the first six months, the period during which the Israeli study found the greatest rate of weight loss. By contrast, the Israeli subjects were 91% male, and fell from an initial dietary carbohydrate intake of 50.8% of total calories to a final value of 40.4%. They were also studied at their workplace, where it seems they were given a great deal of guidance concerning their allocated diet at the main meal of their day.

In summary, what does the data tell us about the modified Atkins-type diets?

Firstly, the diet should ideally not just be low-carbohydrate, but also high in certain fruits and vegetables. Secondly, if the diet is strictly enforced, weight reduction is consistently better than with a low-fat diet, and more rapid than with a calorie-restricted Mediterranean diet. Thirdly, the diet is anti-diabetic, which is logical, as excess carbohydrates strain the mechanisms that regulate the blood sugar. Fourthly, there are only hints—without proof—that this diet reduces heart attacks; neither is there any data that suggests it is good for the brain (Fig. 4.4). In fact, when rats are fed a high-fat diet for only nine days, they suffer from cognitive impairment, according to a recent study from the Departments of Physiology at the Universities of Oxford and Cambridge. Fifthly, in the Israeli study that favoured the Atkins-type diet, the subjects were working males taking their main meal in a cafeteria with fixed food allocations, none of which is very relevant to the enquiring Western-style woman who wants to lose weight, is not externally supervised in her choice and eating of food, and has her main meal in the evening.

Now we need to consider the many other choices of diet.

Low glycaemic index (GI) diets

The principle is that certain foods allow greater absorption of carbohydrate and more rapid rise of blood glucose than other foods do. This sequence elicits a greater need for compensatory insulin release, thereby straining the pancreas and predisposing to diabetes. An extension of the concept is that a low glycaemic index diet may help to avoid the onset of type 2 diabetes, and benefits glucose control in established type 2 diabetes.(11) In theory, then, heart attacks should be lessened. Conversely, a high glycaemic load increased heart attacks by 90% in the large and prolonged Nurses' Health study in the USA.(9)

The big problem is that the list of low GI foods can be totally overwhelming. For example, Foster-Powell in Australia listed 43 pages of products in the *American Journal of Clinical Nutrition* in 2002. Even a more practical but still detailed list of low GI foods is formidable.(12) Thus, I give a simplified outline of the concept: avoid sugar, sweets, potatoes, popcorn, biscuits, cakes, pies, and all the treats that are offered with drinks or tea and coffee. Use olive oil and vinegar in place of sunflower or canola oil. Choose bread that is labelled low GI. It's worth noting that the low GI diet given to diabetics lowered blood levels of the marker of tissue inflammation, C-reactive protein (CRP).

Less inflammation of the coronary artery wall means less coronary disease (see page 50).

For diabetics and pre-diabetics, a simple low glycaemic index diet is logical. I strongly recommend a carbohydrate and calorie-restricted Mediterranean diet that substantially decreases the need for glucose-lowering drugs in newly diagnosed diabetics.(13) Glycaemic control is better than on a low-fat diet, while 'good' HDL-cholesterol is higher and blood triglycerides are lower, so that coronary risk falls.

Other diets

The five-a-day diet

The simplified concept is that eating five items of fruit or vegetables every day will reduce heart attacks, stroke, and possibly cancer. But as far as I could ascertain, no randomized controlled study clinches the idea of the benefit of five-a-day, even for heart attacks and strokes. Rather, five-a-day should be incorporated into the proven DASH or Mediterranean diets.

The DASH diet for high blood pressure

DASH stands for Dietary Approaches to Stop Hypertension, and the DASH diet is high in fruit and vegetables, low in dairy products and fat, low in red and processed meats, low in animal protein, low in sweetened beverages, and low in sodium, but with substantial plant protein from legumes and nuts. It is, therefore, a low-salt, low-olive-oil modification of the Mediterranean diet especially tested in hypertensive people. One excellent long-term study shows that the DASH diet not only lowers blood pressure, but is associated with a lower risk of coronary heart disease and stroke, over 24 years of follow-up.(14)

The South Beach Diet

This diet uses the logic that the glycaemic index (GI) must be kept low to limit the conversion of blood glucose to body fat, and that increased exercise helps to keep the blood glucose down and breaks down tissue fat. The person on this diet often feels good, perhaps partly in response to the cheerful, relaxing name.

The Ornish diet

This diet goes the other way, increasing legumes and high-fibre carbohydrates to allow double the carbohydrates found in the South Beach diet. Cholesterol and saturated fats are strictly limited, so this diet is really low in fat. All animal products are excluded except for egg whites and non-fat dairy products. Thus, this diet may be a good option for vegetarians. Although highly rated according to some criteria, there are no studies so far showing it reduces heart attacks or strokes.

The vegan diet

Diabetes prevalence is low in those who follow a totally plant-based vegetarian diet. In a small study, a low-fat vegan diet improved glycaemic control and cardiovascular risk in diabetics.

Healthy vegetarians and omega-3

Vegetarians cannot obtain omega-3 from fish and should therefore take omega-3 capsules (1000 mg daily of EPA and DHA combined, see Fig. 4.7). There are no compelling data that these capsules should have added omega-6 or omega-9 fats. Because meat is avoided, vitamin B12 is often needed.

The Hay Combination diet

Dr Hay, a New York physician, proposed the food-combining diet in the 1920s. Of the three daily meals, one should have only alkaline, carbohydrate-rich foods; the next should feature protein foods with salads, vegetables, and fruit; and the last meal should have starchy foods with salads, vegetables, and sweet fruit. There have been very few well-designed clinical studies of this diet. In the only one I could find, food-combining gave the same reduction in weight, blood glucose, and blood pressure as a balanced diet, both diets being calorie-restricted. The scientific evidence for the advantages of the Hay diet is virtually non-existent.

The Japanese diet—chopsticks and slow eating

In general, the Japanese are seldom obese, have very long life expectancies, and have a relatively low incidence of cardiovascular disease.

The traditional Japanese diet is high in carbohydrate, being built around rice as a staple food, high in vegetables and fruits, and often includes fish daily. In brief, it rather resembles the Mediterranean diet. However, according to a recent book, *The Chopsticks Diet*, a major benefit of Japanese food culture is the use of chopsticks, which leads to eating small portions and delaying the time it takes to consume the meal. As there is up to a 20-minute delay between the stomach becoming full and the brain realizing that the stomach is full, slower eating means less eating. Indeed, the virtues of eating more slowly have been proven on overweight youngsters whose rate of eating was controlled by a small computer.[15]

What about supplementary dietary fats and oils?

This section tries to clarify which are the ideal supplementary dietary fats, starting with the omega-3 polyunsaturated fatty acids and olive oil. Next I consider those fats of 'mixed qualities' such as canola and sunflower oils. However, I advise against the use of two oils that are very high in saturated fats: coconut and palm oil (Table 4.5). I will also warn against bad fats (including transfats). The most dangerous fats of all are those that are denatured by high temperatures and pollutants as in fast-food outlets.

Technical data on structure of fatty acids

The omega-3 (ω-3) fatty acids are a family of long-chain polyunsaturated fatty acids (PUFAs) that have in common a carbon-carbon double bond in the third bond from the tail-end of the fatty acid (Fig. 4.6). Nutritionally essential are: α-linolenic acid (ALA, 18 carbon), eicosapentaenoic acid (EPA, 20 carbon, Fig. 4.7), and docosahexaenoic acid (DHA, 22 carbon). The human body cannot synthesize omega-3 fatty acids *de novo*, i.e. from scratch, but it can form 20- and 22-carbon unsaturated omega-3 fatty acids from the 18-carbon omega-3 fatty acid, α-linolenic acid (Fig. 4.6). Both the omega-3 α-linolenic acid and omega-6 linoleic acid are essential nutrients that must be obtained from food. Synthesis of the longer-chain protective omega-3 fatty acids from linolenic acid within the body is competitively slowed by the omega-6 structures, as in linoleic acid. Thus, accumulation of long-chain omega-3 fatty acids in tissues is more effective when they are obtained directly from food or capsules, or when competing amounts of omega-6 fatty acids do not greatly exceed the amounts of omega-3 fatty acids.

Table 4.5 Fat content of seeds, oils, and fatty fruit

Substance (seed, nut, oil)	Saturated fat content	Monounsaturated fat content	Polyunsaturated omega-3 content	Polyunsaturated omega-6 content
Example	Palmitic acid, C16	Oleic acid (C18:1, omega-9)	Linolenic acid (C18:3, omega-3)	Linoleic acid (C18:2, omega-6)
Flaxseed	Up to 9%	Up to 19%	up to 80%	Up to 14%
Olive oil-like				
Olive oil (variable)	Up to 20%	Up to 83%	<1.5%	Up to 21.0%
Avocado	20%	70%	0%	10%
Almond	5%	78%	0%	17%
Mixed properties				
Canola (rape seed)	7%	54%	7%	30%
Peanut	18%	47%	0%	29%
Sunflower oil	12%	14–40%; 82% if high	0%	48–74%
Pumpkin seed oil	9%	34%	0–15%	42–57%
Walnut oil	16%	28%	5%	51%
Soybean oil	15%	26%	7%	50%
Evening primrose oil	8%	11%	0%	81%
Avoid				
Coconut	91%	6%	0%	3%
Palm kernel	85%	13%	0%	2%

Major source of data: Udo Erasmus, *Fats that Heal, Fats that Kill*, Alive Books, 1993.

Mixed = variable benefits

C = carbon chain length

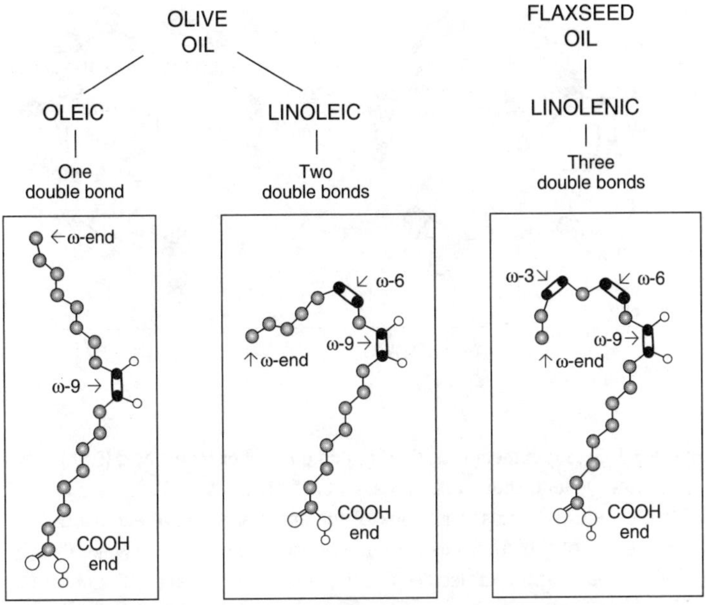

Figure 4.6 Fatty acids: structure of those with an 18-carbon backbone. *On the left* is oleic acid, a normal circulating fatty acid and the chief fatty acid in olive oil (Table 4.5). It is the major fuel for the heart and provides most of the energy needed for cardiac contraction. Oleic acid has 18 carbons (C18) and one central unsaturated double bond (ω-9, counting from the top end). *In the central panel* is linoleic acid, a lesser constituent of olive oil (up to 21%), with a second unsaturated bond in the ω-6 position. In some other oils, it makes up to 80% (Table 4.5). *On the right* is linolenic acid, abundant in flaxseed oil, with three unsaturated bonds in positions ω-3, ω-6, and ω-9. It is the only 18-carbon fatty acid that has the potentially beneficial ω-3 structure, but it requires conversion in the body to 20- and 22-carbon compounds to become the beneficial type of cardioprotective ω-3 fatty acid (ω = omega: the final letter of the Greek alphabet).

For those who find it difficult to follow the Mediterranean diet

To get perfect blood lipids, there are several goals to aim for: low total blood cholesterol, with two components—a low LDL (low-density lipoprotein) and a high HDL (high-density lipoprotein). We have already discussed the two diets (the modified Atkins and the

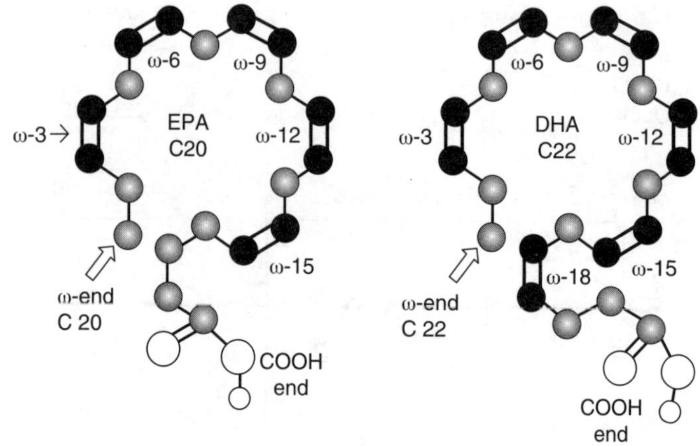

Figure 4.7 Eicosapentaenoic acid (ECA) and docosahexaenoic acid (DHA), two protective long-chain omega-3 essential fatty acids. In ECA there are 20 carbon atoms, one at each kink of the chain and one at each end. Note the site of the crucial ω-3 double bond, three carbons away from the omega (ω) end of the molecule. The five double bonds allow the molecule to flex in on itself, so that it can penetrate cell membranes more easily. In DHA there is an extra double bond so that the chain is two carbons longer. Both are found in fish oil capsules with the ideal being a higher amount of DHA because of its stronger effect on the immune system and on the brain.

Mediterranean) that are better than the low-fat diet of the American Heart Association (AHA). However, even that conservative body has endorsed the use of omega-3 fatty acids for secondary prevention of cardiovascular events in people with documented coronary artery disease. This recommendation marks the first time that the AHA has supported the use of any nutritional supplement for the prevention of cardiac disease. Overall, there is a large and growing body of evidence supporting the cardiovascular benefits and triglyceride-lowering effects of the omega-3 fatty acids.

Combination therapy

Adding omega-3 fatty acids to medication (statins such as Lipitor, Crestor, or simvastatin) is a safe and effective way to improve lipid levels, and to improve estimated cardiovascular prognosis beyond the benefits provided by statin therapy alone. As statins are now increasingly used to lower 'bad' LDL-cholesterol (not only in those who have already had heart attacks, but to prevent heart attacks), and as statins do not act strongly to increase 'good' HDL-cholesterol nor to reduce blood triglycerides, it is a small step to combine statins with a Mediterranean diet, which would achieve both of these aims. This is common-sense advice that I often give. If the diet fails or is poorly adhered to, then omega-3 capsules are the answer.

Omega-3 capsules: what dose and which fatty acids?

Fish oil is widely sold in gelatin capsules containing a mixture of omega-3 fatty acids, including EPA and smaller quantities of DHA. A standard dose of EPA plus DHA is 1000 mg, once daily for established disease such as heart failure and after heart attacks, or double dose for disease prevention. Researchers have found that fish oil high in DHA and low in EPA lowers inflammatory markers (such as the cytokines IL-6 and IL-1β) associated with complex diseases involving neurodegenerative and autoimmune mechanisms. Note that the brain normally contains DHA but no EPA. A high intake of DHA is recommended for pregnant and lactating women, as DHA is essential for the development of the foetal and neonatal nervous system and brain. DHA can also be obtained as a vegetarian product, extracted from algae. Yet another source is krill, a crustacean.

Flaxseed oil (also called linseed oil)

Where could the required very-long-chain omega-3 fatty acids come from, besides oily fish or omega-3 capsules? Omega-3 also comes from flaxseed oil, which contains alpha-linolenic acid (ALA), an omega-3 fatty acid with 18 carbons, the name often shortened to linolenic acid (Fig. 4.6). The body can convert ALA to the beneficial longer-chain omega-3 fatty acids, with 20 (Fig. 4.7) or 22 carbons. Flaxseed oil has two other advantages: first, it is cold-pressed from the seeds, so there is no chemical extraction or modification; and second, it contains lignans, complex chemicals that are oestrogen-like and antioxidant in their action. However, the health-giving properties of lignans have not yet been established beyond doubt. If you choose the flaxseed oil option, remember that it is very susceptible to oxidation induced by light and room temperature. The opaque container must therefore be kept in the refrigerator, tightly closed, and used soon after being opened, not stored.

Which is better as a supplement—flaxseed or fish oils? High quality fish oil contains the two omega-3s that are especially important, the 20-carbon (EPA, Fig. 4.7) and the 22-carbon (DHA) omega-3s, whereas flaxseed oil contains the 18-carbon omega-3 (Fig. 4.6) that must then be converted and upgraded by the body to the 20- and 22-carbon-length compounds. The latter process may be slowed by an excess of omega-6 fatty acids.

Oleic acid and olive oil

Oleic acid is an 18-carbon monounsaturated fatty acid with a double bond in the omega-9 position, found especially in olive oil (hence its name), in high-oleic sunflower oil, in avocados, and in many nuts, including almonds. As a group, the monounsaturated fatty acids increase HDL-cholesterol, which is an important aim in the heart-healthy diet. There is also some reduction of 'bad' LDL-cholesterol and—importantly—decreased oxidation of LDL-cholesterol. These changes imply (but do not directly prove) that coronary disease would be lessened by intake of these fatty acids.

Avocado oil

In general, avocados and avocado oil are likely to have effects similar to those of olive oil (Table 4.5). When avocados are out of season, avocado oil is a good substitute, although it is not certain that the oil contains the 'non-oily' benefits of avocados. For example, avocados also have 60% more potassium than bananas, and are rich in vitamins B, E, and K. They have one of the highest fibre contents of any fruit. Avocados also contain high levels of beta-sitosterol (a beneficial plant-based fat) that reduces the amount of cholesterol absorbed from food. Although the ideal daily dose is not known, half a ripe avocado should be beneficial, at a guess.

Almonds

In high doses (about 75 g per day of unblanched, unroasted, unsalted almonds) almonds can modestly decrease 'bad' LDL-cholesterol and increase 'good' HDL-cholesterol. The most marked effect is reduction of oxidized LDL, which is the form of LDL that is taken up into the coronary artery. The problem with almonds lies in the high doses required to achieve these excellent results, and long-term enthusiasm for such daily doses is seldom kept up.

Mixed quality oils—canola oil and others

These have 'mixed properties'—mixed because some of them resemble olive oil in having high oleic acid contents, but as a group they are characterized by high levels of omega-6 fatty acids (Table 4.5). Canola oil is often used in 'heart-healthy margarines'. Note that in general, some of the industrial methods of extracting oils from the seeds can cause problems. In October 2006, the American Food and Drug Administration (FDA) commented that: 'Limited and not conclusive scientific evidence suggests that eating about 1½ tablespoons (19 grams) of canola oil daily may reduce the risk of coronary heart disease. To achieve this possible benefit, canola oil is to replace a similar amount of saturated fat and not increase the total number of calories you eat in a day.'

The health benefits of omega-6 fatty acids appear to be supported by an advisory review issued in 2009 by the Nutrition Subcommittee of the American Heart Association.[16] Two points are worth commenting on. First, olive oil contains the omega-6 fatty acid linoleic acid (Fig. 4.6), and olive oil is beneficial. Thus there is no question that when omega-6 is coupled with omega-9, as it is in olive oil, there can be no harm; rather, benefit is expected. The problem arises with the very high omega-6 content of oils such as canola. Second, the few beneficial outcome trials that are cited in the American Heart report all focused on replacing saturated fatty acids with omega-6 fatty acids, exactly the same condition for benefit already pointed out by the Food and Drug Administration in 2006.

In simple language, canola is better than an equivalent amount of saturated fat; but must be taken *instead of* and not in addition to the saturated fat.

Sunflower oil

Sunflower oil is difficult to place because several types of sunflower oils are produced, with preparations that vary from high-linoleic sunflower oil, which typically has at least 69% linoleic acid (Fig. 4.6), to high-oleic sunflower oil, which has at least 82% oleic acid and therefore closely resembles olive oil in its properties. However, olive oil can be extracted from olives by cold pressing, without any of the industrial processes required for the conversion of sunflower seeds to oil, so it is a better option.

Omega-3 versus omega-6 fatty acids

Both omega-3 and omega-6 are essential fatty acids, meaning that they cannot be manufactured by the body, and must therefore be included in our overall diet. The optimal ratio of omega-6 to omega-3 is thought to be from 1:1 up to 4:1. These ratios probably evolved during the roughly two million years of evolution of dietary patterns adapted for survival, when sources of omega-3 (such as grass-eating game animals and seafood) were plentiful. This meant there was no need to develop the enzymes that could synthesize omega-3 or omega-6 fatty acids. By comparison, in current Western-type diets, ratios of omega-6 to omega-3 usually exceed 10:1, going up to 20:1 or even higher. So the overall need is to increase omega-3 and to decrease omega-6 fatty acids.

What is so special about fish oil omega-3 fatty acids?

Why are the very-long-chain omega-3 fatty acids beneficial to health? First, they consistently decrease blood triglycerides that, like cholesterol, promote arterial disease, and are licensed for this purpose in the USA and Europe.

Second, they are unsaturated in many sites (polyunsaturated), which allows them to be incorporated more easily into cell membranes, where they have a beneficial influence on the various ion channels (such as sodium and potassium) that open and shut during the wave of electricity that travels over the heart to cause cardiac contraction. These properties explain why omega-3 capsules reduce the chances of dying in heart attack survivors (Table 4.3). By relaxing arteries, they have a modest blood-pressure-reducing effect.

They also benefit the developing brain, where they help to construct the myelin sheaths that protect the conducting parts of the brain cells.

There is also an effect in reducing markers of tissue inflammation, thereby inhibiting a process that contributes to disease of the coronary and cerebral blood vessels. These mechanisms may explain why omega-3 supplementation improved cognitive function in a recent large study (See Chapter 7).

Arachidonic acid

This essential long-chain fatty acid sits at the head of the *arachidonic acid cascade* that normally helps to control a wide range of biological functions, but especially those involving chronic inflammation and blood coagulation. For example, by forming prostacyclin, this cascade inhibits small blood cells (platelets) from clustering together to form blood clots that can block the arteries. This protective anti-platelet effect is similar to that of aspirin. But excess activity of this cascade is undesirable, because it promotes blood clotting and, for some unknown reason, cancer. Being 'essential' but not found in food, this fatty acid must be synthesized by the human body from dietary linoleic acid, as found in high amounts in canola and sunflower oils and to a lesser degree in olive oil (Fig. 4.6; Table 4.5). Thus, diets with excessive emphasis on canola or sunflower or similar oils could pose a threat, whereas the amount of linoleic acid in olive oil seems to be about right.

Transfats

The American Heart Association has become the first big health group to urge a specific limit on transfats in the diet—less than one per cent of total calories—in new guidelines released in 2006. Transfats, more correctly called trans fatty acids, are abnormal in their structure when compared with their normal counterparts (Fig. 4.8). These toxic fats are formed from other fatty acids (such as oleic acid) by heating and reheating, which is what happens in many fast-food outlets. Because transfats cannot be broken down readily, they are stable, and are often inserted to preserve the shelf life of biscuits, pies, bread, cakes, and a variety of packaged or baked foods.

Transfats are even worse for our health than saturated fats, largely because they are foreign to the body and so are not metabolized. They thus accumulate in the body tissues to cause damage. Transfats promote insulin resistance and diabetes, as well as heart disease. They also raise

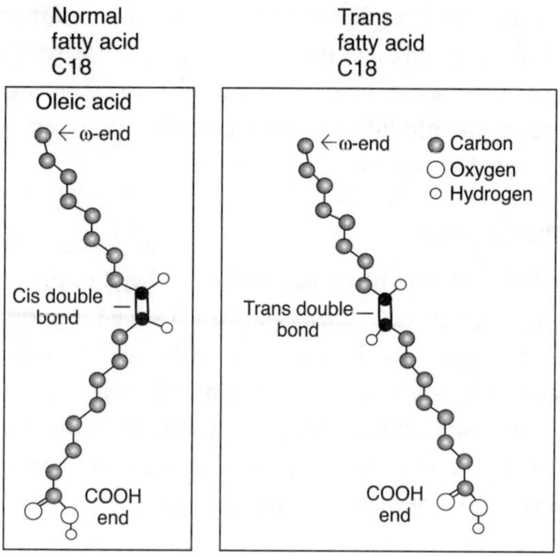

Figure 4.8 Transfat transformation. Oleic acid, on the left, is the normal circulating fatty acid chiefly derived from olive oil (Figure 4.6). It is the major fuel for the heart, and provides most of the energy needed for cardiac contraction. It has 18 carbons (C18) and one central unsaturated double bond (omega-9, counting from the top tail). At the site of the double bond, there are two attached hydrogen atoms, both on the same side of the molecule ('cis' is Latin for 'on the same side'). Because unsaturated fats such as oleic acid have this 'kink' or bend, the molecules do not stack together easily, so that they stay fluid at room temperature and can be broken down in the body. Healthy oleic acid is transformed into unhealthy transfat, shown on the right, through heating. The normal bent cis-form on the left becomes the straightened 'trans' form, which is more stable but toxic to the body because it cannot be broken down ('trans' is Latin for 'on the opposite side', as in transatlantic).

'bad' LDL-cholesterol and lower 'good' HDL-cholesterol, the exact opposite of what needs to happen for good health.

Avoiding transfats

In reading labels, steer clear of 'partially hydrogenated' fats, because these contain transfats. Increasingly, food labels must show the transfat content, making it easier to avoid foods that are bad for our health. Transfats can also be a restaurant hazard, as they are formed from normal fats by repeated reheating. Avoiding them (and sticking to a healthy diet) is challenging when eating out, as many Americans and Europeans do. Avoid fast-food outlets unless they are transfat-free, as they are in France, and now in New York City.

What about the various oil supplements?

Polyunsaturated fatty acids are liquid fats (such as those found in olive oil), in contrast to solid saturated fats (as in butter or red meat) that find their way more easily into the coronary arteries. The polyunsaturated fatty acids contain several double bonds in their fatty acid chain structures, hence the name 'polyunsaturated'. Depending on just where these double bonds are in the fatty acid chain, the polyunsaturated fatty acids are protective against coronary disease.

As a reminder, when the double bond is located on the third site from the tail-end of the chain, it is called an omega-3 bond. This confers cardiovascular protection and is found in fish oils. This bond also contributes to the heart-protective properties of flaxseed oil. For those who have had or are at high risk of heart attacks, I recommend added omega-3 capsules. These have much better supporting data than any other oil supplements.

Practical advice when buying health supplements

Omega-3

When you consider purchasing health supplements, remember that only one has clear evidence in its favour: omega-3 fish oil capsules with a total dose of EPA plus DHA of 1000mg. Go to a supermarket rather than a 'health shop'. You will have more freedom of choice and may feel less pressurized. Look carefully at the label; there should be a detailed list of the fatty acid composition, specifically stating which of the fatty acids the capsule contains. There must be a line in the label stating 'contains no transfat'. The need for omega-3 capsules can be avoided—albeit at a cost, but with a gain in pleasure—by regularly eating oily fish. My personal choice is wild salmon, which is low in mercury (Table 4.4). Flaxseed oil should also work, but there is a lack of clinical data to show that it lessens heart attacks. Use it as a dressing for salads when you need a change from olive oil. Both oils mix well with balsamic vinegar.

When it comes to other supplements, none have evidence strong enough to be compelling. Regarding margarines, again there is no decisive clinical evidence to guide your choice, and I regard canola, with its high omega-6 content, as one of the fatty acids of 'possible but unproven virtue'. Why not just be Mediterranean and dunk your bread (carefully chosen or homemade) in olive oil and balsamic vinegar, and ditch the butter and margarine?

Can drugs be used instead of diet?

By far the most common drug used to control obesity is nicotine, which exposes us to the risk of displacing one addiction (to food) with another. The amphetamines and similar substances in nicotine promote nervous system activity. Again, addiction is a real problem, with the added risks of increased probability of heart attacks, stroke, lung cancer, and other serious illnesses. Almost all models use nicotine this way, regardless of the risks, with the result that, for instance, one supermodel developed emphysema at age 31—this despite having given up cigarettes five years previously. There are prescription drugs that are much safer, and that help the patient to achieve weight loss at the same rate that would result from a strict diet (Table 4.6).

Orlistat interferes with the gastrointestinal absorption of fat, and has a proven long-term effect when added to a weight-reducing diet. In one study, it prevented the progression from obesity to diabetes, the latter being a feared complication of obesity. It may have gastrointestinal side-effects such as flatulence and diarrhoea.

Sibutramine acts as an adrenergic stimulant, which (like exercise) breaks down fat tissue, but at the cost of a slightly increased heart rate and blood pressure.

Rimonabant inhibits the cannabinoid receptors, the newly discovered brain receptors that are stimulated by cannabis. The cannabinoid receptors are associated with pleasurable impulses such as appetite for food and smoking. This drug has a potential double effect, reducing both the desire to eat (and thus weight) and the desire to smoke. Unfortunately, it has adverse psychiatric effects on mood as it dampens the pleasure responses. This has caused serious mental depression in a minority of patients, with a few cases of suicide reported. This drug is presently available in Europe, but is restricted to very few

Table 4.6 Comparative effects of diet and drugs on parameters of obesity and diabetes

Diet/Drug	Wt loss kg	Glucose mmol/L	HbA1c	BP mmHg	LDL-C mmol/L	HDL-C mmol/L	TG mmol/L	Side-effects
Atkins modified	–4.7	↔	↓0.9%	↓3.9/0.8	–0.08 (–3.0 mg/dL)	+0.22 (8.4 mg/dL)	–0.27 (–24 mg/dL)	↔
Mediterranean, 'HMS Healthy'	–4.4	–1.8; (–33 mg/dL)	↓0.5%	↓5.5/2.2	–0.14 (–5.6 mg/dL)	+0.17 (6.4 mg/dL)	–0.25 (–22 mg/dL)	↔
Low-fat	–2.9	↔	↓0.4%	↓4.3/0.9	–0.001 (–0.05 mg/L)	+0.17 (6.3 mg/dL)	–0.03 (–3 mg/dL)	↔
Orlistat (Xenical)	–2.9	–1.0	↓0.4%	↓1.5/1.4	–0.26	–0.03	–0.03	GI
Sibutramine (Reductil)	–4.2	↔	↔	↑1.7/2.4	–0.03	+0.04	–0.18	Adrenergic
Tesofensine† (0.5 mg plus diet, exercise)	–9.1	–0.11	↓0.08%	↑0/1.5	↔	+0.04	–0.24	Nausea; Adrenergic: HR↑7.4
Rimonabant	–4.7	–1.0	↓0.7%	↓1.8/1.2	–0.05	+0.10	–0.24	Psychiatric
Liraglutide†† **(Vitoza)** By injection; subcutaneous	–7.2 (max dose) –6.3 (3.0 mg dose)	–0.44	↓0.24%	↓6.9/2.9	NS	NS	NS	Nausea; reduced BP; prevented pre-diabetes in obesity

HbA1c = haemoglobin A1c, an index of blood glucose levels over 24 hrs; BP = blood pressure; LDL-C = low-density lipoprotein cholesterol; HDL-C = high-density lipoprotein cholesterol; TG = triglyceride; GI = gastrointestinal; HR = heart rate.

HMS = *Harvard Medical School Guide to Healthy Eating*, Willett WC et al., New York, Simon & Schuster, 2001.

↔, unchanged values; NS = not significant; L = litre

†Astrup A, et al. Lancet 2008; 372: 1906; ††Astrup A, et al. Lancet 2009; 374: 1606

selected patients. It is not available at all in the USA, where registration was refused.

Tesofensine is a drug in development that acts by inhibiting the reuptake back into the nerve terminal of the stimulatory nerve system messengers, noradrenaline, dopamine, and serotonin—one of the processes used in psychiatric antidepressant therapy. Of the doses used, 0.5 mg for an average weight of 100 kg gives the greatest weight loss with tolerable side-effects (insomnia, dry mouth, nausea, constipation, and fast heart rate), and is associated with improved physical function and self-esteem.

Liraglutide and exanitide are registered antidiabetic drugs that inhibit appetite, leading to weight loss. They must be given by injection, daily for liraglutide and weekly for exanatide, hence are best for diabetics or for pre-diabetics. Furthermore, nausea is a major albeit transient side-effect.

Because of the difficulties, dangers, and cost of using drugs to lose weight, the quest for weight loss basically comes back to sticking to a sensible diet and exercise. However, prescription drugs may support the battle for weight loss in selected cases.

Summary and recommendations

Overall, weight loss must start with the grit and steely determination to stick to the chosen diet. Among a plethora of diets, an intelligent understanding of why a specific diet is chosen is helpful, as is group therapy. I'm impressed by the potentially rapid initial weight loss seen with the modified Atkins-type diet, as in the Israeli study; this encourages the overweight person or cardiac patient to carry on dieting.

After this initial phase of a few months, I recommend switching to the Mediterranean diet, in the absence of long-term health outcome studies of the modified Atkins-type diet. Apart from the Mediterranean diet, I could find little or no information on what impact long-term adherence to any other diet has on the incidence of heart attacks, strokes, or cancer, or what effect it has on longevity and brain function.

The Mediterranean diet (really an eating pattern) is far superior in its established long-term health benefits. As emphasized, it is easy to

Table 4.7 Five key ways to protect heart and brain

1. How to lose weight (NB: expect limited sustained loss up to 6 kg):

Step one. Build up determination to stick and to succeed. Choose the diet best suited to your needs. If undecided, start with the modified Atkins diet and increase daily exercise.

Step two. After achieving weight loss, at about four to five months, swap to the Mediterranean diet for long-term health and heart protection. Continue with exercise and calorie restriction.

Step three. Long term, the major problem is how to stick to the diet (adherence). My advice: interactive group discussions and group exercise.

How to remember the Mediterranean diet: The five-H mnemonic: High vegetables, High fruit, High fish, High olive oil, and a Handful of nuts every day.

2. How to fix blood cholesterol:

LDL 'bad' cholesterol decrease:

Dietary: Avoid animal fats, butter, and hard cheese. Modified Atkins or Mediterranean diets are beneficial.

Exercise: In adolescence† not in adults.

Drugs: If needed, especially statins such as Lipitor or Crestor; also niacin or fibrates.

3. HDL 'good' cholesterol increase:

Dietary: Modified Atkins or Mediterranean or low-fat diets.

Nuts: Almonds; some other nuts.

Exercise and weight loss.

Alcohol: Moderate.

Drugs: If needed—niacin, fibrates, glitazones, trimetazidine (statins, weak effect).

4. How to decrease blood glucose:

Simplified low glycaemic index diet and vigorous exercise.

5. How to decrease BP and protect brain:

Weight loss and low-salt Atkins diet.

Then swap to DASH diet or low-salt Mediterranean or add olive oil to DASH.

Then consider medication.

6. The only proven cardioprotective supplement; memory may improve:

Only one supplement gives documented cardioprotection—omega-3 capsules.

Mechanisms complex; include significant reduction of blood triglycerides.

Alternative: oily fish.

†Kelley GA. Atherosclerosis 2007; 191: 447.

simplify the Mediterranean diet to a five-H mnemonic: High vegetables, High fruit, High fish, High olive oil, and a Handful of nuts every day. However, calories *must* be restricted to maintain weight loss.

Overall, for the long-term, if you overlook the lack of good health outcome data, you can take your pick of any of the diets, according to what you find easiest to stick with and which of them best suits your needs and lifestyle. In my view, the crucial issue is one of willpower—to initiate the diet of your choice, and then (most difficult) to stick to it.

Bottom line

My overall dietary advice is summarized in Table 4.7. I list five major aims: weight loss; a good cholesterol profile (low 'bad' LDL and high 'good' HDL-cholesterol levels); low blood glucose; low blood pressure; and high omega-3 intake. If that is too complex, adhere to the five-H mnemonic. Make a point of eating 'all the colours every day' when choosing fresh vegetables and fruit.

If all else fails, the simplest advice is: eat more slowly, and do more exercise—you may lose some weight, and you'll feel much better.

Chapter 5

Fads vs. Facts

Can excess antioxidants actually hasten your demise?

Since 'everyone knows' that supplemental antioxidants can protect the heart and blood vessels from damage, and many still think that the antioxidant vitamin tablets (vitamins A, C, and E) must be beneficial, how can I ask such an outrageous question? The burning issue is whether these antioxidant vitamins can reduce coronary heart disease. Closely related is the claim that antioxidants help to preserve brain power. Enthusiasts who take antioxidants claim reduction of coronary disease and cancer with better brains to boot. This chapter summarizes the data that dispute these claims with special reference to coronary heart disease and discusses why antioxidant vitamins that should work don't do their job as they should. It is often thought that antioxidant vitamins and folic acid protect from heart disease (Table 5.1). Rather, some promote harm. I will suggest that natural antioxidants, such as in the Mediterranean food pattern, are the best way to take truly protective antioxidants. Thereafter I discuss the water craze, green tea, calcium tablets, and hormone replacement therapy.

Antioxidants: what are they?

Antioxidants are substances that protect against oxygen free radicals. These are highly unstable forms of oxygen with an extra electron, which gives the name 'oxygen free radicals' (technically shown as •O2- in Figs. 5.1 and 5.2). Free oxygen is highly interactive and potentially toxic, yet when present in normal amounts carries crucial messages that are essential for the heart and blood vessels to function normally. Note the contrast between potentially adverse free oxygen radicals

Table 5.1 Do antioxidant vitamins and folic acid protect from heart disease?

Vitamin type	Dose	Outcome benefit/harm
Mixed, from food	Mediterranean diet has mixed normal antioxidants	Fewer heart attacks and strokes; longevity
Vitamin A (beta-carotene)	High dose	Promotes cancer or is neutral
Vitamin C	Low–medium dose	Modest protection from common cold
	Dietary protection High dose, pro-oxidant	Optimal dose 100 mg/day High dose damages DNA
Vitamin E (alpha-tocopherol)	High dose in multivitamins	No benefit, some mortality harm
Folic acid	High dose supplements	No benefit to heart, harm if coronary artery disease; memory benefit (controversial)

formed in the body and the stable oxygen molecules that we inspire and are then carried from the lungs by the blood, eventually to be converted into energy by all living body cells. Thus the oxygen in the atmosphere, if unpolluted, does not poison us.

Oxygen free radicals: 'right ROS' versus 'wrong ROS'

Oxygen free radicals are physiologically protective but in excess potentially dangerous. Confusingly, they are now often called Reactive Oxygen Species (ROS), which it must be stressed are part of the normal body's defence mechanisms. ROS are physiologically produced in the mitochondria during conditions of normal blood supply with normal oxygen delivery. I call these protective molecules 'right ROS' (Fig. 5.1) because low levels promote cell growth, whereas high levels promote cell death. **Right ROS** are also a crucial part of the messenger system that partially protects the heart from a heart attack, especially when treated by opening up the blocked artery. In that situation the oxygen radicals are part of the complex chain of events that can minimize the

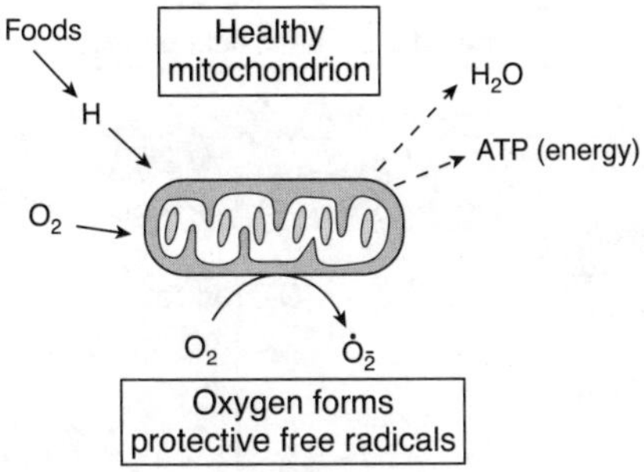

Figure 5.1 Right ROS (Reactive Oxygen Species). In normal, healthy cells small amounts of these oxygen free radicals are formed by mitochondria, the power houses of cells, converting oxygen and hydrogen (left side) to water and energy in the form of ATP (adenosine triphosphate, right side). These modest amounts of oxygen radicals are protective and required for normal cell growth. Thus high doses of antioxidants, as in many supplements, may lessen the formation of this required amount of oxygen radicals and inhibit protective functions. © Opie.

problems caused by the sudden return of blood to the damaged tissue. However, when there are too many oxygen radicals around then they become damaging because they kill cells and need to be opposed. **Wrong ROS** (Fig. 5.2) may damage more than the heart, and can for example experimentally promote cancer-like changes in various body cells. Thus, there is a very delicate balance between the right and wrong amounts of the active radicals of oxygen.

Keeping the oxygen balance

To keep this balance between the beneficial and harmful effects of oxygen radicals, nature has evolved antioxidants found in food and, what is more, found in the right amounts. Of all the diets, those high in fruit and vegetables and low in processed foods and transfats, as in the traditional Mediterranean diet (Chapter 4), are most likely to keep at bay excess free radicals. The potentially harmful effects of high doses of antioxidants, taken as supplements, can be visualized as the situation where not only are the harmful free radicals wiped out, but so are the beneficial ones. But which are the antioxidant vitamins involved? These are vitamins A, C, and E, of which vitamin E has received most attention.

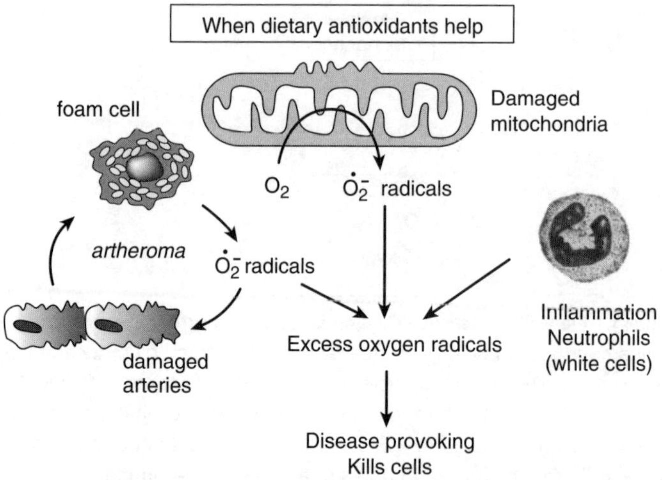

Figure 5.2 Wrong ROS. Excessive amounts of oxygen free radicals are harmful. Three major sources are, from left to right: first, in diseased coronary arteries oxygen radicals are formed from foam cells, which contain the cholesterol deposits (Fig. 2.4); second, diseased mitochondria form excess oxygen radicals; and the third source is white cells that are increased in states of tissue inflammation, now known to be an important process in the development of coronary artery disease (Fig. 3.8).© Opie.

Population versus properly randomized controlled studies

The hope of antioxidant benefit comes from what are called observational studies of the distribution of disease in the population (epidemiology). For example, in 79 542 subjects a high dietary vitamin E intake was associated with a 37% reduction in cardiovascular mortality, as published in the leading medical journal, *The Lancet*, in 2001. One of several observational population studies in postmenopausal women found that those with the highest dietary intakes of vitamin E had a 58% reduction in the risk for coronary death, whereas there was no benefit of dietary vitamin A and C.

The major problem in interpreting observational studies lies in what are called *confounding factors*, such as socioeconomic and lifestyle factors. For example, those naturally taking a high vitamin E diet (high fruit and vegetables) could also be those who are more health conscious and better exercised. Take another example. Years ago, in South Africa, when the great American epidemiologist Ancel Keys first found the relation between blood cholesterol levels and coronary disease, those people with coronary disease living in Cape Town (and elsewhere) were much more likely to be eating a high-fat, unhealthy diet. But they were also wealthier and had more telephones. An observational study would have incorrectly suggested the possibility that the mere act of having a telephone would increase the risk of heart attacks.

Which are reliable trials?

Such confounding (in simpler terms: confusing) factors can to some extent be allowed for by 'corrective calculations' (also called adjustments) but adjusted data are not as valid as well-designed prospective controlled trials that compare the agent or drug under test with a matched dummy (placebo). There must be clearly defined end-points such as deaths or heart attacks or strokes or cancer. Such studies are randomized, properly controlled, and give definitive trustworthy results, especially because both doctors and patients are 'blinded', meaning that neither party knows which tablet is active and which is the placebo.

Blinding is essential because there is a well-established placebo effect whereby dummy tablets can improve symptoms and even partially seem to reverse the disease process, probably acting by psychological mechanisms. Thus the active ingredients must perform better than the dummy to give a trustworthy result. In contrast, observational studies are 'hypothesis generating', meaning that they raise a proposal to be tested (such as vitamin E supplements are protective) but must be followed by proper prospective trials that are needed to give proof of cause-and-effect. In the case of vitamin E, the observational studies suggest cardioprotection whereas the prospective well-controlled studies show no benefit or even show harm. But how can studies on, let us say, coffee drinking be made 'blind'?

Harsh reality—risks of synthetic vitamin E and other antioxidants

In a *Lancet* 2004 study on 170 000 people taking vitamin pills, cancer was not prevented and death rates were increased by 29% in those taking both beta-carotene (a form of vitamin A) plus vitamin A supplements, and by 10% in those taking beta-carotene plus vitamin E. In an even more telling and recent document, a very careful meta-analysis of 68 randomized trials with antioxidant supplements and with 232 606 participants in no less than 385 publications, there were the following startling findings in the *Journal of the American Medical Association* in 2007.(1) The end-point was very simple—mortality. If antioxidant supplements really made a difference, they would alter mortality. Taking together all the trials, there was no effect on mortality. However, when taking the trials that were best designed ('low bias risk'), in 180 938 participants the antioxidant supplements increased mortality, albeit by only 5%. Beta-carotene increased deaths by 7%, vitamin A by 16%, and vitamin E by 4%.

Vitamin E remains the biggest sinner because it is the most popular antioxidant bought as a supplement and is consistently found in multivitamin preparations. In usual doses found in multivitamins, 400 or more units per tablet, vitamin E does not benefit those at risk of heart disease or cancer, including diabetics, as shown by the very large study by the excellent group at McMaster University.(2) The Editorial in the same issue concluded that this study 'effectively closed the door on any major protective effect of this supplement in moderately high doses', referring to cardiovascular disease.

Vitamin E and memory

Vitamin E is also often thought to protect against cognitive decline (the fancy term for memory loss with age). In a well-designed study, long-term use of 600 units on alternate days over 9.6 years by generally healthy older American women failed to improve cognitive function. Would even higher doses help? In those with mild cognitive improvement, a daily dose of 1000 units was increased to 2000 units after six weeks for a total of three years, without any improvement in memory, as published in the *New England Journal of Medicine* in 2005. Indeed, such high doses may increase all-cause mortality.(3) Mortality started to increase as the daily vitamin E dose increased above 150 units per day, whereas doses of 400 units are common in supplements.

No wonder that the Johns Hopkins group urge health professionals to warn the public 'against the use of ineffective or even harmful interventions, such as vitamin E, that may compete with well-established preventive measures. High-dose vitamin E is a prime example of misplaced priorities.'[3]

Vitamin C and other antioxidants

Logically, based on many epidemiological observational studies, dietary supplementation by other antioxidants (vitamin C, beta-carotene, selenium, zinc) should reduce cardiovascular disease and cancer. However, vitamin C can act both as a pro-oxidant and as an antioxidant. Vitamin C in doses above 500 mg daily promotes adverse changes in human DNA, according to a paper in the leading research journal *Nature.*[4] This dose is common in supplements, and higher megadoses are available with the idea of 'megaprotection'.

Overall, the data with Vitamin C are controversial. There have been no large well-designed prospective outcome studies. Two observational dietary studies found a reduced cardiovascular disease risk as vitamin C increased, with an optimum at about 100 mg per day, but one other study goes the other way. There is modest protection against the common cold.

Vitamin A

The dietary precursor of vitamin A, beta-carotene, promoted lung cancer in a large Finnish study. In a pooled analysis of eight studies on 138 113 participants, deaths due to all causes rose modestly by 7% in the beta-carotene group, as reported in *The Lancet* in 2003. This finding is very serious for an agent that is supposed to promote health. Men who have a low plasma beta-carotene level are more likely to develop hypertension. However, beta-carotene supplementation had no effect on the risk of developing hypertension in a group of French men. Indeed, the results were resoundingly negative. Overall, there is no good evidence that multivitamin supplements reduce cancer except in badly nourished Chinese populations, according to an expert panel reporting in the *Annals of Internal Medicine* in 2007.

Natural antioxidants in the Mediterranean diet: what you eat matters

What is clear and would explain the epidemiological studies is that a diet high in fruit and vegetables provides the right amount of the various antioxidant vitamins in the correct balance between them. The Mediterranean diet is an example. It is high in fruit, vegetables, and olive oil, but low in red meat and saturated fats, and often goes with red wine (for details see Chapter 4). Both high quality green olive oil and red wine are high in antioxidants. Very convincingly, the greater the adherence to this diet, the higher the total antioxidant capacity of the blood.[5] Furthermore, this diet with plentiful green leafy salads, also called foliage, provides more than enough folic acid (see later in this chapter).

What should work versus what works

Thus, there is a puzzling difference between what *should* work and what *does* work. Many epidemiological studies show that those who have high dietary intakes of antioxidants have less cardiovascular disease. Yet there is no clear-cut evidence that supplementary antioxidants work, and good data for harm. This conclusion relates to the apparently healthy people studied. This does *not* mean that patients who are seriously ill cannot benefit from supplements. In those who are seriously ill and at nutritional risk, such as with severe heart or kidney failure, the situation is different and benefits of vitamin supplements may be found.

Thus, for the average apparently normal person there is no evidence that vitamin E supplementation improves the health of the heart, nor lessens the risk of developing some dreaded diseases like Alzheimer's, nor protects from cancer. Rather there is potential for harm for the majority of those who buy the high doses available at 'health shops'.

Vitamin E: explanations for the difference between facts and the enthusiasm of 'health workers'

Beauty is in the eye of the beholder, and so it seems is the evidence for vitamin E. Despite the overwhelming negative data on vitamin E in prospective randomized trials available even in 2001, the Harvard epidemiologists Willett and Stampfer concluded that vitamin E supplements are 'reasonable' for Americans at risk of coronary disease, in their article 'What vitamins should I be taking, doctor?' in the highly influential *New England Journal of Medicine.* Maybe the new negative data in 232 606 people (yes, over one-quarter of one million people) in the randomized controlled trials summarized by Bjelakovic in 2007[(1)] should make apparently well-educated Americans and Europeans think more critically and clearly about vitamin E supplements.

Why is it that vitamin E supplementation that should work, not only does not but could harm? First, oxidative stress has a hypothetical role in the pathogenesis of many chronic diseases, but it might be the consequence rather than the cause of these conditions. Second, oxidative stress may benefit rather than harm the heart by clearing away dying cells (apoptosis), scavenging foreign bodies (phagocytosis), and by detoxification. Third, antioxidant supplements are synthetic and not subject to the same rigorous efficacy and toxicity studies as pharmaceutical agents that are approved by bodies such as the Food and Drug Administration (FDA) in the USA.

Fourth, in the hierarchy of evidence, observational studies rank lower than well-designed large prospective randomized trials in which the drug or supplement is given and compared with a placebo to assess effects on predetermined outcomes such as death or heart attacks. These trials are double-blinded, meaning that neither the patients nor the doctors know who is receiving the active treatment. Such prospective intervention studies with vitamin E show zero effect on mortality with a modest increase in deaths in the best designed trials.[(1)]

Fifth, and the explanation that I like best, is that the molecular form of vitamin E found in supplements, namely alpha-tocopherol, has a harmful structure despite its antioxidant effects. The form of vitamin E actually found in the natural diet is gamma-tocopherol,[(6)] which I call 'Good E'. In the circulation, large doses of vitamin E supplements in the alpha form compete with the natural Good E (gamma-tocopherol) for binding sites on the blood proteins, thereby displacing the Good E and decreasing its protective effects. The blood levels of Good E are low in patients with coronary disease, and Good E is about twice as powerful in preventing oxidation of 'bad' (LDL) cholesterol as is the alpha form. These little known facts can at least in part explain the failure of high-dose vitamin E supplements to provide benefit against disease.

Hypothesis: Good vs Bad E

Thus an important hypothesis derived from all the available data is that there is a potentially protective role for dietary but not for supplemental vitamin E. The Nutrition Committee of the American Heart Association recommends diets high in antioxidants without giving population-wide recommendations favouring vitamin E supplements because of the absence of efficacy and safety data from randomized trials. If vitamin E were presented to the Food and Drug Administration in the USA, would it achieve a licence for anything? Resoundingly, the realistic answer is 'no'. By contrast there is clear evidence for protection by the Mediterranean diet, and in many large studies for those with hypertension by licensed drugs such as the angiotensin converting enzyme (ACE) inhibitors or calcium channel blockers, or for those with too much 'bad' (LDL) cholesterol by the statin drugs such as Lipitor and Crestor.

Flavonoids and flavonols

'Dark' is the flavour of the month, it seems. The word 'flavonoid' means dark in colour and embraces a large number of compounds, including those found in intensely dark chocolate, dark cocoa, and red wine. In general, the flavonoids improve the function of the inner layer of the arterioles, where they enhance the production of vasoprotective nitric oxide and decrease oxidative stress. These qualities can be tested in the laboratory. For example, cocoa rich in flavonol, the active ingredient in flavonoids, has an effect like nitric oxide that induces dilation of the forearm arteries in healthy humans and dilation of the coronary arteries in transplant patients. Of interest, the active agent of the flavonol-rich cocoa is the natural antioxidant epicatechin, also found in red wine and olive oil.

Does this mean that we should all be adding some dark chocolate to our evening meals? First, as pointed out in an important editorial by Dr Norman Hollenberg from Harvard that explores the underlying mechanisms, the word 'dark' is a misnomer. For chocolate, there is no strict relation between colour and flavonol content; the actual content should be printed on the wrapping paper.(7) Theoretically it is possible to have high flavonol white chocolate. Furthermore, consider what is added to dark chocolate. There is 11 g of sugar and 18 g of fat for a 40 g serving of the very dark chocolate (where one square variably equals 5 to 6 grams). The sugar and fat may have adverse effects on the many people prone to diabetes or metabolic syndrome, about 40% of the population, or those prone to coronary disease, probably about 20% of the population, with higher figures for India. Chocolate is often made up with milk and milk itself inhibits some of the benefits of chocolate. Logically, dark chocolate with more flavonols should be more protective than milk or white chocolate.

Headlines versus original reports

Judging by the enthusiastic newspaper headlines, all doubts about the beneficial cardioprotective qualities of chocolate have been removed by a careful prospective study published in the *European Heart Journal* in March 2010. The headlines said that the benefits were confirmed and that only modest amounts such as one small slab of the bar were protective. Some papers said dark chocolate now had the OK. Nearly 20 000 Europeans were studied over eight years. Those who ate only an average of 7.5 grams of chocolate (where 50 g = one bar) had almost 40% less heart attacks and stroke than those who only nibbled an average of 1.7 grams per day. The presumed mechanism was BP reduction, but the measured BP only fell slightly. The chocolate was mostly milk, not dark, which is important because milk may interfere with the beneficial action of flavonols. Common sense questions whether small amounts of flavonol-poor chocolate could do such wonders or whether self control in eating so little chocolate was a marker of general health consciousness. That such small amounts of flavonols could really give benefit remains to be established in the future by proper randomized trials.

Can small amounts of flavonols really give health benefits?

Daily doses of only small amounts equal to one square (6.3 g) of very dark chocolate decreased the BP modestly after 18 weeks but only by 2.9/1.9 mmHg (systolic/diastolic values). This BP lowering effect of very dark chocolate was not found in matching flavonol-free white chocolate.[8] How did the dark chocolate work? By increasing blood levels of nitrate compounds, which are similar in structure to the nitrate drugs given into the bloodstream by doctors when rapid reduction of BP is needed in an emergency. Yet in these very low doses, the amount of BP reduction is hardly significant. Rather, to achieve substantial BP reduction of say 5–11 mmHg, would need 100 g of the very dark chocolate with 50% cocoa daily, which would bring with it about 480 calories. This is about 20 to 25% of the normal daily calorie needs. As pointed out in the June 2010 issue of *Hypertension*, sponsored by the American Heart Association, the risk is that of sustained weight gain, which (as discussed in Chapter 4) might well have many other serious health consequences, probably including an increase in blood pressure. Careful large and long-term studies are needed to settle these issues.

Nonetheless, the principles are clear—flavonols are beneficial. Right now, what it does mean is that there is hope, at least in the longer-term future, that there will be a dark chocolate without dark side-effects such as weight gain. In the meantime, modestly indulge or drink cocoa.

The folic acid mystery: another paradox

While some years ago it was fashionable to treat mild elevations of homocysteine in the blood with folic acid, in several large studies the data now show that there is no cardiac benefit to be found when outcome studies are undertaken. Heart attacks are not reduced. Indeed, one study suggests that folic acid has adverse effects in those with coronary disease.[9] Why, if an increased blood homocysteine is associated with a greater risk for coronary disease, does bringing it down by using folic acid supplements not give benefit? This is called the 'homocysteine paradox'.[10] One current explanation is actually very simple: the elevated blood homocysteine results from kidneys that are not working perfectly. They fail to excrete enough homocysteine and it builds up in the blood. However, this homocysteine increase is harmless. The real problem is the underlying incipient renal disease, often clinically missed, that gives rise to elevations of truly noxious substances in the blood. Seen in that light, modest elevations of blood homocysteine are no direct marker of cardiovascular disease, but rather a marker of renal disease that, in turn, is causing or promoting the cardiovascular disease.

Other more complex explanations are proposed by Dr Joe Loscalzo, Chief of Internal Medicine at the Brigham and Women's Hospital of Harvard Medical School, to explain the 'complex reasons' why in the case of homocysteine the clearly negative trial outcome results conflict with the theoretical benefit that should have been found. In an Editorial in the *New England Journal of Medicine*, the world's leading medical journal,(11) he suggests that excess folic acid hinders the formation of protective nitric oxide. Another important point is that folic acid is a growth factor that promotes cell growth and may do so in the lipid plaques of the coronary arteries, which would explain why folic acid supplementation caused increased blockage of stents in one study.

Not yet the end of the folic acid story

Of course pregnant women need enough folic acid to avoid defects of the nervous system in the foetus. There are other factors too that are keeping the folic acid hypothesis alive—one being that folic acid supplementation is legally required in cereals in North America, and might provide just enough and not too much folic acid. Indeed, in two major studies on a total of 39 005 subjects, folic acid combined with vitamins B6 and B12 very modestly reduced stroke in countries outside of North America where there is no folic acid fortification.(12,13) In the Vitamin Intervention for Stroke Trial, this same folic acid combination could not prevent stroke.

Of interest, despite all the many negative or borderline controlled trials, the folic acid hypothesis still lives on, especially in relation to the brain and vitamin B therapy (see page 154).

For those readers who seriously wish to prevent stroke, be sure that your blood pressure and cholesterol patterns are such that you do not need blood pressure or cholesterol reduction, both of which give clear reductions in heart attacks and strokes in large trials. If you are experiencing cognitive loss and already taking high-dose omega-3 capsules, try high dose vitamins B12, B6, and folic acid (see page 154). Omit folic acid if you have heart problems (page 101).

Other vitamin supplements

In general, informed public opinion has veered against vitamin supplements since the publication at the end of 2008 and start of 2009 of a series of negative well-designed placebo-controlled studies on the lack of effect of vitamins C and E on heart attacks, stroke, and cancer.[14,15] Yet another study showed that beta-carotene had no effect in preventing lung cancer. These very large studies come from a group at Harvard Medical School who are leading investigators in these very reliable studies. In another excellent study from the University of Texas, selenium did not prevent prostate cancer. Altogether these studies covered nearly 40 000 men followed for 5–8 years.

Of course the negative studies on males exclude any benefit of supplements in prevention of breast cancer in females, as claimed in a recent study from Puerto Rico that hit the headlines as 'Calcium, vitamins can save women'. What the headlines do not say is that this was only a small study based on a self-administered questionnaire among Puerto Rican women whose initial health status was not established. Nor do the newspapers report the comment from the American Cancer Society that 'the totality of evidence does not support taking vitamins and calcium' in normally and adequately nourished women.[16] To realistically assess your risk of breast cancer, Google the US National Cancer Institute.

Nor do negative studies on well-nourished people exclude benefit in those who might have borderline health. For example, the Chinese prevention trial reported reduced total cancer by 13% by using very much lower doses of vitamin E, selenium, and beta-carotene than in the American studies, which used the usual high doses available in 'Health Shops'.

What about the remaining vitamin B components as supplements? In the well-designed Norwegian Vitamin study (NORVIT), in those who had already suffered from heart attacks there was a trend towards more repeat attacks in those who received vitamins B6, B12, and folic acid. Note that in this well-nourished population, the folic acid in green leafy vegetables would already have provided enough folic acid and that more could have been an overdose for the heart.

What about multivite tablets?

From the evolutionary perspective, our ancestors developed their metabolic patterns on a diet of wild fruit and vegetables, supplemented by fish and meat, rather than being adapted to large doses of specific vitamins. Most multivitamin preparations simply contain far too much of each vitamin. Another problem is that vitamins often need interaction between each other and co-factors to be fully active. Overall, a mixed diet rich in fresh vegetables and fruit is most likely to deliver optimal doses of the various vitamins.

Other supplements

These are many, and the major point is that well-designed trials with proper outcome studies are few and generally negative (see Chapter 7 for Gingko biloba). A problem with newspaper reporting is that when the negative supplement trials come out, they constitute 'no news' and therefore miss the public eye. *Overall, vitamin supplements for the heart have the potential for harm contrasting with the modest benefit conferred by some (Fig. 5.3).* For the brain, see page 154.

Fluid fads: water, sugary drinks, and coffee

Dr Bernard Lown, winner of the Nobel Peace prize and an experienced cardiologist and promoter of healthy lifestyles in the holistic therapy of the cardiac patients who attend his Boston-based clinic, has tackled the 'water craze'. He writes in his online journal ProCor: 'I was taken aback when an elderly patient confessed dejectedly that she didn't drink the eight glasses of water her physician had prescribed. I was astounded to learn that water loading for all comers pervades medical practice. But how robust is the scientific evidence and how did this come about? A systematic search of the medical literature turned up a blank.'

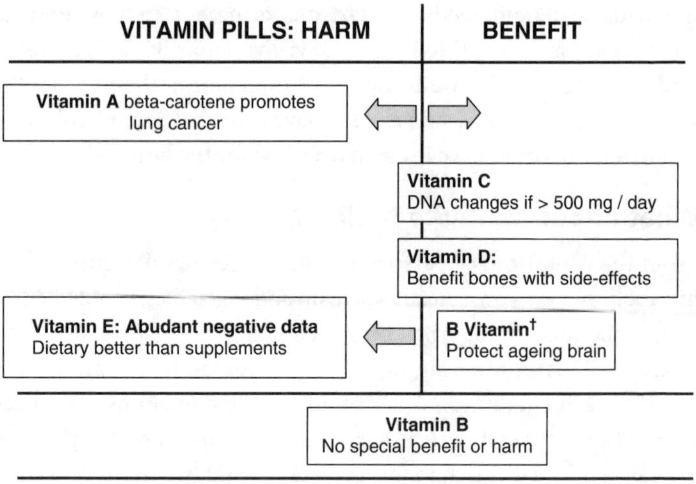

Figure 5.3 Variable benefit or harm. There are few vitamin preparations that benefit people who are in apparently good health and eat normally. Increased calcium intake is required as age progresses but should not be overdone†. See page 154. © Opie.

'The minimum daily requirement of liquid has been defined. Those residing in moderate climates lose about 500 ml or 16 American ounces of water daily. This is referred to as the obligatory fluid loss, and includes water mandatorily excreted by the kidneys and the insensible water loss from skin through evaporation. Such losses are readily replaced by the high content of water in solid food and by the fact that most people consume beverages such as coffee, tea, fruit juices, wine, and alcohol.'

'Is there any benefit though from additional fluid intake?' asks Dr Lown. 'No scientific evidence supports the greater efficacy of dieting when water intake is increased. Nor does water dosing combat kidney stones, urinary tract infection, or bladder cancer. How did binging on water come about? In fact, I do not know. Aggressive beverage marketers like Coca-Cola and PepsiCo are more likely suspects. In the short span of a few years their water brands became blockbuster successes. The current market for bottled water is huge and growing. A variety of factors drive demand. Topmost in my view is the erroneous view that we are prone to dehydration unless constantly replenished.'

How much water should I drink a day?

This is a simple question with no simple scientific answer. So what is Dr Lown's response? First, a sense of thirst controls fluid intake very well unless there is serious disease. If a number must be given to counter the eight glasses per day, then 250 ml of liquid (eight American ounces) with a meal should suffice for those not running a marathon or living in the tropics. Tap water is fine, and in most industrialized countries is bacteriologically and environmentally superior to bottled water. I might add that for those who enjoy wine, Dr Lown's 250 ml per meal corresponds to one-third of a bottle of wine, or roughly two drinks per day at dinner, with its own benefits. Personally, I still enjoy lightly sparkling bottled water with a restaurant meal. Dr Lown's advice can be found on his website at http://www.procor.org/advocacy/advocacy_show.htm?doc_id=697463.

Sugary soft drinks

These tend to be taken by two classes of people. First, those already obese and at increased risk of diabetes, such as African American women, who are particularly prone to being overweight and obese. Those regularly consuming two or more sweetened fruit drinks or soft drinks were more likely to develop diabetes by 37% or 50% respectively. These results probably also apply to other obese women. As diabetes is a dread disease, the message is not only to avoid excess calories but to cut out such soft drinks, which should be replaced by water and other healthy fruit drinks such as orange or red grapefruit juices.(17)

Young people aged 14 to 25 are the other group increasingly vulnerable to soft drink advertisements that promote the health-giving picture. Leading the way is the USA, then Germany, and then France. For them, there is likewise the danger of future diabetes, but clear statistical data are not available.

Coffee and tea

When I was on sabbatical leave at Stanford University in California, it was striking how much coffee was drunk all day by one and all. For most people, coffee stimulates the adrenaline nervous system to accelerate waking up and has the same effect throughout the day with repeat doses. However, any benefits of coffee were thrown into doubt when early studies showed that caffeine (an important component of coffee) when given acutely interferes with the use of glucose by the body with the potential risk of inducing diabetes. Caffeine but not coffee enhances physical performance.(18) Some components of coffee block certain effects of caffeine, so that the two cannot be equated.

Surprisingly, and through ill-understood mechanisms, in long-term population studies coffee decreases the risk of diabetes and might reduce total mortality with a suggestion of a dose-related benefit.(19) A Dutch population study over 10 years found that three cups of coffee were able to stem, to some extent, the dread cognitive decline (loss of memory).(20) The mechanism may be similar to the stimulatory effect of nicotine on memory. However, coffee can't cure all. In the study by the Harvard School of Public Health, who followed up a large number of American health professionals and nurses for 14 years, increased coffee drinking of up to six or more cups per day had no apparent effect on coronary heart disease,(21) but in the same study was linked to modest stroke reduction in women. None of these studies show any clear cause and effect relationship. Of note, there may be important lifestyle and economic differences between the coffee drinkers and others. In summary, there are no data strongly suggesting that much coffee drinking is harmful, and some to suggest a protective or memory-enhancing effect. Thus it is difficult to criticize all those Stanford academics and their coffee craze.

Green tea and the Asian paradox

In Japan, China, and other Asian countries, it is a social custom to drink green tea, which is less processed, made from unfermented tea leaves, and richer in antioxidant catechins. The so-called 'Asian paradox' is the lower than expected rate of deaths from coronary disease and lung cancer. The Food and Drug Administration (FDA) of the United States has previously stated that green tea probably does not reduce breast, prostate, or any other type of cancer. Nonetheless, the belief that drinking green tea confers health benefits has driven up its popularity over the last decade, according to the Tea Association of the United States.

The Japanese company that bills itself as the world's largest green tea company, and its US subsidiary, petitioned the FDA in June 2005, seeking to make the claim that drinking at least five ounces of green tea a day may reduce the risk of heart disease. However, the FDA carefully reviewed 105 articles and other publications submitted as part of the petition but could find no scientific evidence to support claims of the beverage's health benefits. The FDA concluded that there is no credible evidence to support qualified health claims that green tea or green tea extract could reduce any of the risk factors associated with cardiovascular disease. (A health claim, in the language of the FDA, characterizes the relationship between a substance and a reduction in the risk of contracting a particular disease.) Rather, it seems to me, the lower than expected rate of coronary disease, for example in the Japanese, may be explained by the high amounts of oily fish in their diet. For green tea and memory, see page 166.

Calcium

Osteoporosis may have no direct relation to the health of the heart and brain, but a bent back dents the self-image, which indirectly detracts from the cardiovascular benefits of a healthy lifestyle. As age progresses and the bones naturally thin, most women start taking calcium supplements to prevent bone thinning (osteopenia in a mild form and osteoporosis in a severe form with a high risk of bone fractures). About 1200 mg per day increases bone mineral density (the bones thicken) both in postmenopausal women and in older men, the latter not studied until recently.[(22)] Vitamin D 400–800 international units is added to ensure adequate uptake of calcium. In the largest trial, which lasted for seven years and involved apparently healthy postmenopausal women of average age 62 years, there was a 29% decrease in hip fractures. This, however, translated into an absolute decrease of only four fewer hip fractures per 10 000 women, somewhat offset by a 17% increase in kidney stones.[(23)] Increased weight-bearing exercises should improve the bone results.

Added to the risk of kidney stones, researchers from New Zealand wrote in the *British Medical Journal* in January 2009 that they found increased heart attacks in their postmenopausal women treated by calcium given as 1000 units per day. These women had a high level of exercise and a very low level of smoking, but were still at increased risk of heart attacks because of their seriously high cholesterol values (6.73 mmol/L, versus an ideal of less than 5.0 mmol/L). Presumably they had succumbed to the large amounts of high quality, high-fat dairy products and red meat readily available in that country. Prudent advice is to get the cholesterol and 'bad' LDL-cholesterol to desirable levels before embarking on calcium supplements. None of these studies report on a simple issue: did those who took the calcium plus vitamin D supplements have straighter backs with less drooping?

Can the best diet for the heart, the Mediterranean diet, also prevent osteoporosis? Three components are associated with increased bone density: plenty of fish and olive oil with little red meat.[(24)] The issue of calcium supplements must be decided by the estimated risk of fracture in each person; for example, thin, smoking women definitely need calcium and vitamin D. A practical tip: if you decide after evaluating the data and consulting a good doctor that calcium plus vitamin D really is for you, then calcium citrate rather than the usual calcium carbonate will cost much more but should remove the risk of kidney stones.

Hormone replacement therapy (HRT)

Clinical trials of postmenopausal hormone replacement therapy (HRT) have shown increased risk of coronary heart disease (CHD) in the first few years after initiation of therapy and no overall benefit. Those with higher levels of low-density lipoprotein (LDL) cholesterol, and hence in any case at greater risk of CHD, were at further risk of CHD when given HRT.[(25)] The best bet is to calculate the expected cardiovascular risk in any given woman and then to multiply that by about one-third to get the effect of HRT in increasing the risk (Gaziano risk table for women, Fig. 3.5).

A female with a low risk, as many modern women are at the menopause, won't have much increase in the absolute risk rate. For example, a calculated 10-year risk of cardiovascular disease of say 5%, then increased by a further expected 33% due to HRT, would have a risk of

6.7%, which could be offset by tighter lipid or blood pressure control. In practice women are now increasingly advised to take HRT for a few years after the menopause and then to tail it off.

Doctor, what do you take?

As I am on a Mediterranean diet, happily consuming fish, olive oil, red wine, and many green folic-acid-containing vegetables, I am vitamin replete and only take what else is essential. In my case, I take vitamin B12 because with age my blood B12 has fallen and my red cells have grown larger, and these are corrected by B12. Such minor degrees of B12 deficiency often develop with age. If left untreated, long-term and significant B12 lack can impair mental function and interfere with the sense of position of the legs. I also take calcium (not carbonate) and vitamin D3 to help to drive the calcium into the bones after careful assessment of my spine.

Summary

Overall, some vitamins and supplements are beneficial, while others have no benefit or are harmful (Fig. 5.4). Antioxidant vitamins E and C, though widely promoted by the 'health' industry, have not stood the test of large reliable trials when compared with dummy (placebo) tablets. The reasons are complex but my suggestion is that oxygen in the free radical form (which means that the molecules are highly reactive) has natural protective functions that are obliterated by the large antioxidant doses in the supplements at the doses in which they are marketed. Regarding folic acid, although there are clear relations between increased homocysteine blood levels and cardiovascular disease, and added folic acid decreases blood homocysteine, yet supplementary folic acid does not decrease and may increase cardiovascular disease. Again, the mechanisms are complex and not easy to understand but the facts are clear. The role of folic acid in stroke prevention is also not clear, being borderline or modest at best, unlike the clear effect of blood pressure reduction.

A new study supports high dose vitamins B12, B6 and folic acid to lessen brain shrinkage with age. I caution against high dose folic acid in those with heart problems.

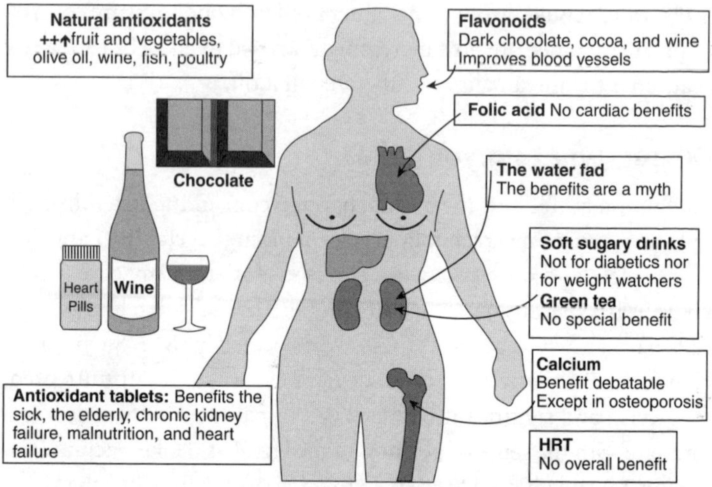

Figure 5.4 Fighting disease by supplements? Not many supplements give true benefit, even though Americans spend more on supplements than on approved medications. Red wine and dark chocolate are natural products, as are the natural antioxidant components of the Mediterranean diet (top left). Both wine and chocolate must be taken in moderation. To avoid the calorie-mediated weight gain that outweighs any benefit of delicacies, daily doses of wine are only 1–2 glasses for women, 2–4 for men, and chocolate is also limited to achieve the flavonoid benefit.

Another unexpected fact is that the need for eight glasses of water per day has no known scientific basis. Sugary sweet drinks are anything but healthy. Coffee drinking even in high doses might well be modestly protective through mechanisms that again are difficult to understand. Green tea tastes well and is proposed to explain the so-called Asian paradox, but the claim of protection from heart disease was turned down by the American Food and Drugs Administration (FDA). Calcium and vitamin D supplements do thicken the bones, but only have modest power in preventing fractures, at least in the American and Australian populations studied. Calcium carbonate carries some risk of increased kidney stones. Careful assessment of bone health is best before embarking on calcium-vitamin D supplements. Otherwise, supplements are not needed for apparently well people taking a healthy diet high in fruit and vegetables. In those chronically and seriously ill, supplementary vitamins come into their own.

Chapter 6

Mind over Matter

Stress, blood pressure, and heart attacks

"The power of the made up mind is critical. When William the Conqueror landed in England, he drilled holes in all the ships. So he had no way of getting back to France. He made up his mind that he was going to take England."
Lewis Pugh, Arctic swimmer and author of Achieving the Impossible

What takes human beings to the limits of their endurance? How did Scott and his team of explorers battle their way to the South Pole? How does a small bird manage to fly across an entire ocean? What enables an Olympic athlete (one who is not using performance-enhancing drugs) to keep doing better and better? How were some individuals able to endure the horrors of the Holocaust?

What is the mind?

While the brain is a concrete organ, with definite activities in its different parts, the mind is a more nebulous concept. The mind refers to a combination of emotional and intellectual activities, often with the implication of intense focus—think of the phrase 'put one's mind to it'. To be in two minds is to be undecided. It certainly does not mean a double brain. Even in Shakespeare, the word has many different meanings. In Coriolanus, he describes a 'mind so rare'. The elderly King Lear feared that he was not 'in perfect mind'. More recently, in 1986, the Royal College of Psychiatrists in London was warned of the twin dangers of 'mindlessness and brainlessness'[(1)] without defining the mind, which has many meanings (Table 6.1). I will take 'mind' to mean that part of the personality that governs and influences the

Table 6.1 Definitions of the mind, based on the *Concise Oxford Dictionary*

1. The seat of awareness, thought, volition, and feeling
2. Attention, concentration
3. The intellect, intellectual powers
4. Remembrance, memory
5. Way of thinking or feeling
6. Focus of one's thoughts and desires
7. Normal mental functioning

emotional life, epitomized by the phrase: mind over matter. For the mind to be active, there must be a functioning brain (no brain, no mind). The mind can both protect from disease and cause disease.

In this chapter, I probe some of the mysteries of the human mind, not just to answer questions like those at the start of this chapter, but to see if the answers hold a clue to better health for all of us. Perhaps we hold the key to curing chronic diseases in our own brains. Is it possible that we might be able to 'cure' our own bodies of diseases like high blood pressure and obesity, and to prevent killers like stroke and heart attack?

These are not easy questions. The theories that try to explain how extreme physical fatigue halts exertion are particularly complex, so here I'll focus on one principal aspect: the mechanisms that set our limits of physical endurance. Is there perhaps a central circuit or switch in the brain that keeps the body going, in spite of other factors limiting the strength and staying power of our muscles?

And on the other hand, we know that psychological stress can limit the way our bodies perform—both in the short term, and by triggering or worsening self-promoted 'lifestyle' diseases such as strokes, heart attacks, and high blood pressure. And this means it's critical to ask how we should be handling stress. Let's not forget that stress (and the illnesses it can cause) can have positive benefits when it triggers changes in habits or lifestyle—chest pains can lead us to ditch the cigarettes, eat more fruit and vegetables, take up walking or cycling, even adopt a pet—all of which will have overall beneficial health effects.

And this leads in turn to two more important questions: when should we turn to medication to manage stress (or conditions such as anxiety and depression caused by stress)? And can the circuits in our brain that monitor pleasure and pain—the 'reward circuits'—be adapted or 'trained' to change behaviour patterns that aggravate stress and stress-related illness?

The vasomotor centre—control room for your heart

Stress is often 'felt' as a fast or irregular heartbeat. How do the impulses that control this change travel from the conscious brain to the heart? At the base of the brain, where the 'thinking' parts are perched on the more primitive part (known as the mid-brain), lies the centre that controls the heartbeat and the opening and closing of the arteries. This is the vasomotor centre, and this is where the signals are generated that make your heart beat faster or slower and your blood pressure rise or fall (Fig. 6.1).

It makes sense that there should be a strong subconscious regulation at work; otherwise, every time you fell asleep, you would have to consciously instruct the centre in the brain to send out impulses to slow down your heart and decrease your blood pressure. Subconscious regulation is essential, and life-prolonging. Why? Because your heart needs to rest and recuperate from the ravages of the day, and your blood pressure needs to be reduced to allow the arteries to restore daytime damage to the endothelium, the thin inner layer of the blood vessels that normally keeps cholesterol out of the wall of the artery.

It's easy to understand how regular exercise can prolong our lives—it promotes a slower heart rate and lower blood pressure. But we don't directly control those effects. So what power can the *conscious* brain exert over the vasomotor centre, and what are the possible consequences?

Overcoming fatigue by the central positive feedback loop

As we know, messages from the conscious cortex can increase the heart rate. For example, earthquakes increase both the heart rate and blood pressure (Fig. 6.2). Earthquakes in California are regularly associated with small but significant spikes in the local death rate. The loud noise and physical shock of the earthquake transmits itself to

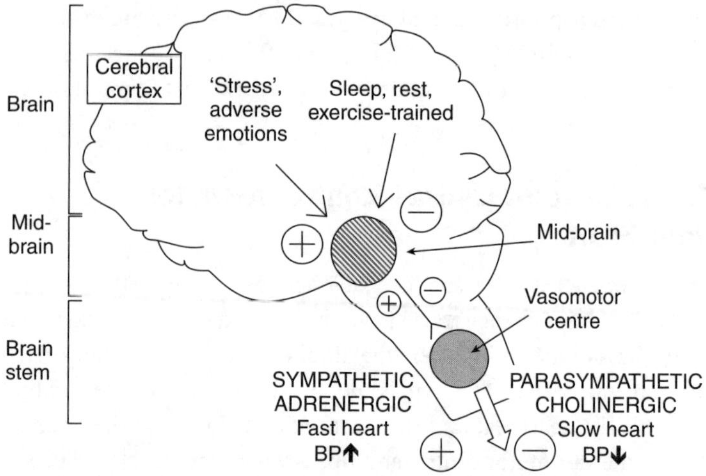

Figure 6.1 The hierarchy of command. Impulses start in the conscious brain, the cerebral cortex, and are then sent 'downwards' to the mid-brain, and from there to the vasomotor centre. Stimulation of this system starts with emotional stimuli, anticipated exercise, and/or psychological stress. From the vasomotor centre, the impulses travel to the heart and arteries to stimulate the heart rate and constrict the arteries (with an increase in blood pressure). Alternately, when the cortex is subject to calming influences such as rest or sleep or after exercise training, the impulses sent out from the mid-brain and from there to the vasomotor centre travel along the parasympathetic cholinergic anti-adrenergic system to send impulses along the vagal nerve to slow the heart and to drop the blood pressure. (Note: the mid-brain contains the specialized part, the hippocampus; see Fig. 6.9.) BP = blood pressure. © Opie.

the vasomotor centre in the lower brain; this in turn stimulates the system to send out nervous impulses that act by releasing adrenaline-like ('adrenergic') messengers at the nerve terminals in the heart or arteries, stimulating the receptors that increase the heart rate and blood pressure. So from this observation and many others, we can draw the conclusion that impulses from the higher centres in the cortex of the brain can stimulate the adrenergic-sensitive part of the vasomotor centre.

But suppose the stimulated vasomotor centre could send signals *back* to the higher centres in the cortex? This reverse stimulation could

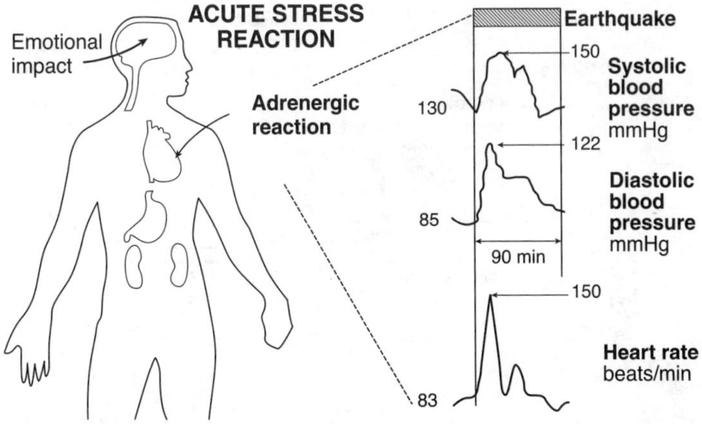

Figure 6.2 An earthquake. Stress, blood pressure, and heart rate all increase at the start of a monitored Japanese earthquake. Data from Parati G, et al. Hypertension 2001; 38: 1093. © Opie.

trigger a beneficial and self-perpetuating cycle that could help overcome fatigue by putting the adrenergic system into high gear so as to give optimum stimulation to the heart and muscles (Fig. 6.3). Here's how it might work:

1 The conscious cortex, the thinking part of the brain, signals it is 'ready to go'.

2 That signal stimulates the adrenergic control centre in the lower brain, which increases the blood pressure and heart rate.

3 Simultaneously there is a reverse 'upward' stimulation back to the cortex…

4 … which then signals it is 'ready to go' again.

An exercise-promoting cycle has been initiated, with the result that fatigue is delayed.

The idea of this emphasis on the role of the brain in controlling the onset of fatigue stems from the 'central governor' theory of Professor Tim Noakes, an international leader in Sports Medicine.(2) Previously, it was believed that the sensation of fatigue arose in the muscles being used, not in the brain. Of course, muscle fatigue can't be eliminated by brain power, only delayed; Scott's expedition reached the South

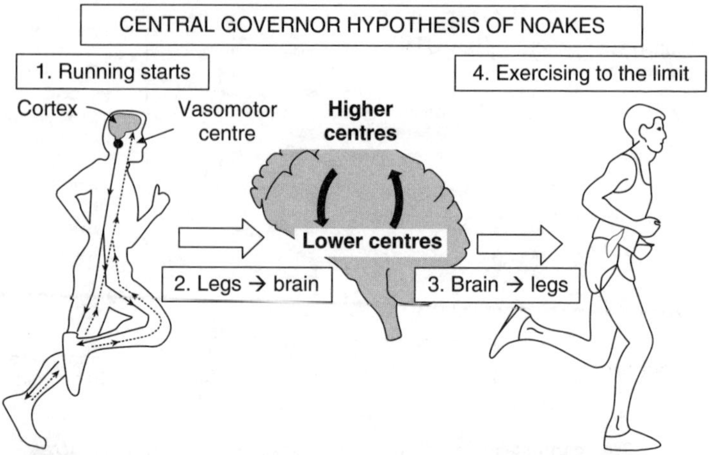

Figure 6.3 The limits of physical endurance. How the mind can influence the body to even greater physical exertion. This phenomenon can be explained by the 'central governor theory' of Professor Tim Noakes, a former colleague and a world leader in Sports Medicine. Step 1 is the initiation of exercise by an act of volition in the cortex of the brain, which sends impulses to the vasomotor centre (Fig. 6.1) and then to the limbs, instructing them to 'start up'. Step 2 is the rapid transmission of signals up to the brain, where the higher and lower centres interact to reinforce each other. Step 3 is the enhanced drive from the brain to the leg muscles. The 'central governor' may be explained in part by the interaction between the higher and lower centres in a manner similar to a 'reward circuit' (Fig. 6.9). © Opie.

Pole, but could not struggle all the way back. Scott's party man-hauled their sleighs across the Antarctic for 159 days. They reached the South Pole and almost made it back, only to die 318 km short of their base camp. Over the course of this ordeal each member spent an estimated 900 000 kcal, certainly 'at the limits' of human endurance.

Control malfunction: stressful anxiety and how to damp it down

As much as the adrenergic system can be spurred to reach the limits of human endurance, it's equally likely that this same system could act harmfully—for example in excessive and prolonged anxiety states. In such cases of hyper-anxiety, the adrenergic input from the cortex is excessive and destructive, and the feedback system now perpetuates a harmful situation, doing still more damage.

Logically, such anxiety should be caught at the source—in the cortex of the brain—by appropriate psychotherapy, or anxiolytic drugs that lessen the anxiety. But psychotherapy is time-consuming and expensive, and drugs have side-effects. When a doctor is confronted by a patient with anxiety and a heart that's beating too fast, sometimes it's simpler just to block the effect of the anxiety on the nerves going to the heart.

Technically, the drugs that can do this are called beta-adrenergic blocking drugs; they block the effect of the adrenaline system on the heart rate, and are more commonly known as beta-blockers. The prototype was propranolol (available commercially as Inderal) and was invented by Sir James Black and published in a premier medical journal, *The Lancet,* in 1962. For this outstanding achievement he was awarded the Nobel Prize. Beta-blockers physically lessen or stabilize fast or irregular heartbeats; the psychological effect is reassurance for those who suffer from anxiety. By showing that the heart is still normal, a major source of anxiety is reduced.

Does stress cause high blood pressure?

Stress is often thought to be the major factor causing high blood pressure (hypertension). If this is true, we could say that stress limits the physical performance of the body, in that it promotes a common disease in which blood pressure is sustained at abnormally high levels (Table 2.1). Several lifestyle and genetic factors interact to sustain high blood pressure levels. If you have a genetic tendency towards high blood pressure, there are several other factors that could make the situation worse: a high-salt diet, weight gain, diabetes—and stress itself. The present chapter focuses on the role of stress in hypertension, but to get the big picture take a glimpse back at Chapter 2.

It is common knowledge that acute psychological stress can cause abrupt increases in blood pressure and heart rate; for example, during an earthquake (Fig. 6.2), or when doctors visit patients in hospital (Fig. 6.4). (This temporary rise when blood pressure is taken by doctors or nurses is known as 'white coat hypertension'.) But blood pressure can shoot up even without the presence of doctors or nurses—my

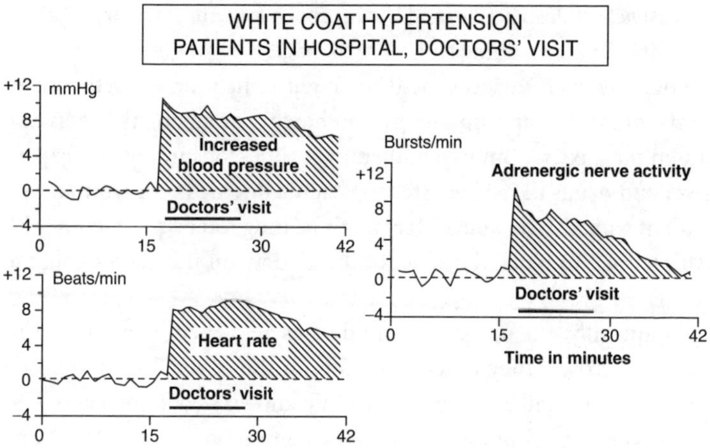

Figure 6.4 'White coat' hypertension. The stress-induced increase in blood pressure and heart rate, associated with increased adrenergic nervous system activity, was caused in this case by the visit of a group of doctors to the patient in hospital. Modified with permission from Fig. 2 of Grassi G, et al. Muscle and Skin sympathetic nerve traffic during the 'white coat' effect. *Circulation* 1999; 100: 222–225. Copyright © American Heart Association.

own blood pressure was substantially higher at the start of a series of measurements I took on myself on an automated recording machine than it was later in the process.

Even if such intermittent stress-related increases in blood pressure are only temporary, over many years, frequent episodes may slowly damage the delicate, sensitive inner layer of the arteries. The result is that your arteries become constricted, and the heart must pump harder to send blood through these narrowed pipes. The increased force of the strongly contracting heart could drive your blood pressure up almost permanently, and this chronically sustained high blood pressure (hypertension) increases the risk of a stroke or heart attack. As if the physiological effects weren't enough, stress may also lead to unhealthy habits such as alcohol abuse, smoking, overeating, and under-exercising—all of which can also raise your blood pressure.

The link between stress and high blood pressure is well known to researchers; mice develop hypertension when they are stressed by being forced to compete vigorously and persistently for access to food or water, or for a safe place to live. A similar example in humans is stress-induced high blood pressure found in those who live under aircraft flight paths near airports, or who experience excessive noise at work. So there is strong evidence that stress is one of several factors that can cause hypertension. But how often does stress cause stroke—especially in those in whom hypertension is not a factor?

What is the real risk of stress-induced blood pressure increases?

Four significant studies have shown that stress increases the risk of stroke. In Finnish men whose details were tracked for 11 years, the magnitude of stress-induced surges in blood pressure at the start of the study was linked to an increased risk of stroke in later life. In a large study in Denmark, involving 12 574 people over 13 years, those who reported that they had high-intensity stress had almost double the incidence of fatal stroke.(3) In an even larger study, 20 627 stroke-free people (two-thirds of whom had normal blood pressure) living in Norfolk, England, completed a questionnaire that measured well-being and psychological stress.(4) After eight and a half years of follow-up, it was shown that stress had increased their risk of stroke by 11%. Thus stress can predispose to stroke, even in those with normal blood pressure.

Note that in these large population studies, the question asked was whether stress could be a major factor in causing stroke—nothing to do with blood pressure. But in the Danish study, the most intense stress levels were associated with greater degrees of hypertension. Conclusion? Stress and significant hypertension go together, and if you suffer from hypertension, ideally you need to control both stress and blood pressure. Often, it is much easier to treat just the blood pressure.

Does anti-stress therapy really treat hypertension?

Despite a period of enthusiasm for yoga and related techniques, practising and expert hypertension doctors have largely lost interest in psychological therapy and relaxation techniques. The reasons are simple. The effects of stress relief on blood pressure have been variable at best, and drug treatment of hypertension has become simple and effective. Many busy hypertensives just don't have the time to learn and to apply stress therapy. And a major problem in managing stress in hypertension is that people under chronic psychological stress often have associated physical and other abnormalities: obesity, lack of exercise, and lack of willpower regarding food and drink—all of which can increase blood pressure—and therefore need treatment.

But we shouldn't make the mistake of relying only on drugs and throwing every stress-relief technique out with the bathwater; surprisingly, stress may be lessened by simple but beneficial lifestyle changes:

- Exercise-induced stress relief is one example. In the Danish study mentioned above, the highest levels of stress were associated with a low level of physical exercise (less than four hours per week). Rearranging your daily programme to include at least 30 minutes of exercise can work wonders.
- Counselling is another simple step to take. If you and your spouse/partner have been trapped in the same argument for years, enlist someone to help you discuss your marital problems.

These measures need to be combined with careful blood pressure control; it's a very good idea to find an expert medical doctor with an active interest in hypertension.

An unexpected example of the impact that life changes can have was seen in a study of highly stressed Wall Street stockbrokers.(5) In that study, stockbrokers who adopted pets found it far easier to blunt their stress-induced blood pressure surges. One of them said: 'Having this pet makes me better able to see what really is important, and to put things into perspective.' The reason? Well, the advantage pets have over people in providing social support is in their non-judgemental nature; they accept their owners unconditionally, which is just what the stockbrokers needed. Thus, another simple lifestyle change:

- If you're highly stressed and hypertensive, get a dog.

Though it may seem obvious, it's surprising how few people are aware of what their blood pressure is under any set of circumstances, so this points to another important way we can control our health:

- Know the enemy: not for nothing is untreated hypertension known as the 'silent killer'. We should all know our blood pressure, and the principles of its management (Table 2.1).

So a stressful lifestyle may promote hypertension—in part indirectly, through excessive drinking or gaining weight. But the direct mechanisms are more elusive, and may work through transient episodes of high blood pressure, which lead to arterial damage. In our modern, stressful society, some react more adversely to stress than others. In blood pressure management, the emphasis should be on tight control, both by way of lifestyle and by the use of drugs. How do we approach this rationally?

You are the best judge of how stressed you are. Your level of stress can be self-diagnosed. If you are one of the minority of hypertensives who react intensely to stress, you should benefit from relaxation techniques. In a few selected stressed people, psychotherapy may be needed. Exercise training reduces stress-induced increases in blood pressure by promoting the activity of the cholinergic blood pressure-lowering nervous system (Fig. 6.1). Perhaps the simplest overall lifestyle advice to counter stress is: take your blood pressure. Talk about it. Then go running with your dog.

Questions that remain about stress and blood pressure

Will beta-blockers, which lower blood pressure by inhibiting the stress-activated adrenaline (USA usage: epinephrine) system, be beneficial for hypertensives who are badly affected by stress? Can stress-induced blood pressure surges be eliminated completely? To date we have yet to see a good trial to test these hypotheses.

At present, all we can say is that obvious stress should be relieved in whichever way is most appropriate for the patient. And while the patient's drug therapy is tailored to their needs, other lifestyle measures such as increased exercise, weight loss, and diet will be very important.

The mind, heart rhythm, and coronary disease

Stress and sudden cardiac death

Although difficult to prove scientifically, it appears there are strong links between stress that invokes adrenergic nervous system activity by the release of adrenaline and noradrenaline, and the severe heart rhythm irregularities induced by anger. This suggests that sudden death could also be evoked by emotional stress (Fig. 6.5). It is especially likely when an individual has significant disease of the coronary arteries; in cases like these, severe emotional stress could be the trigger for sudden total irregularity of the heartbeat (known as ventricular fibrillation), which may lead to cardiac arrest unless the sufferer is revived instantly. Severe emotional stress really can kill, as commonly believed and embodied in the phrase: 'he died from a broken heart'.

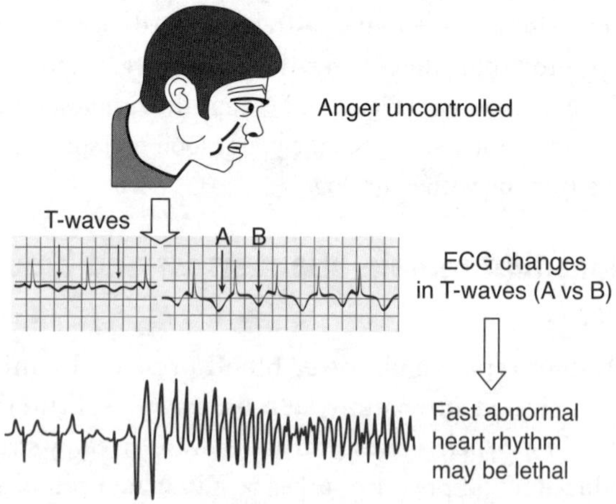

Figure 6.5 Anger causing irregular heartbeats. The electrocardiogram (ECG) pattern shows sudden onset of severe irregular and fast heartbeats in the lower panel, with risk of sudden cardiac death. An early change while the heart rhythm is still regular lies in the changing pattern of part of the ECG pattern called the T-wave. Compare wave A with wave B in the upper panel. (For role of anger, see Lambert R, et al. J Am Coll Cardiol 2009; 53: 774; for ECG changes, see Schwartz P, et al. Am Heart J 1976; 89: 45.)

Mental stress, chest pains, and angina

Stress can generate chest pains likely to make you think you're having a heart attack. (It's also possible that the sudden increase in stress caused by coming to this conclusion could result in a genuine heart attack.) There are important differences between such pain and true cardiac pain that is caused by narrowed coronary arteries (Fig. 6.6). True cardiac pain is called angina of effort, as it usually occurs during physical exertion. It's short-lived, and is an indicator of serious disease of the coronary arteries. In contrast, an aching or stabbing pain directly over the heart itself that is long-lasting is usually associated with anxiety or stress, and isn't related to physical effort. The treatment for

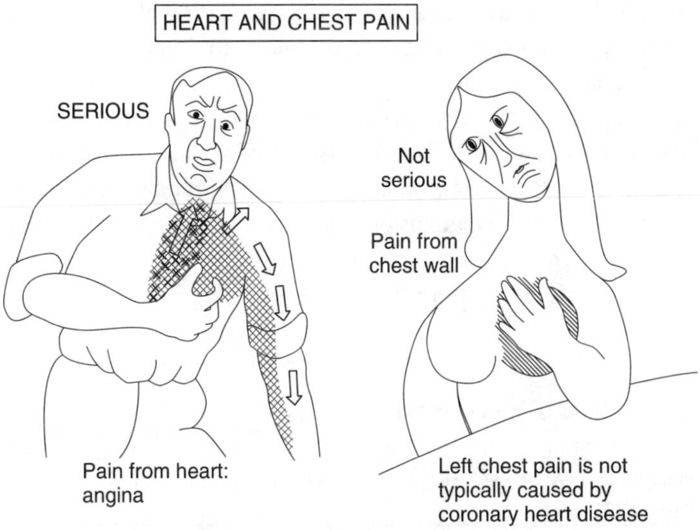

Figure 6.6 Two contrasting examples of chest pain. The typical pain of angina is caused by exercise in the presence of serious narrowing of the coronary arteries. As shown on the left, the pain starts as a tight central pressure in the middle of the chest, which then spreads to the neck and left shoulder and arm. The pain stops the exercise, whereupon the pain fades. On the right we see the pain that originates in the chest wall, not in the heart. It is typically felt directly over the heart, below the breast, for hours and even days. A man is shown on the left because men are more prone to coronary artery disease. Although a woman is shown on the right, the condition was initially described in World War I as 'soldiers' heart'. © Opie.

this 'false' pain is thorough investigation of the patient's history and careful examination of the heart, which will often establish that significant heart disease may be excluded. This type of 'normal' result usually reassures most patients to the extent that the pain goes away, although some will need prolonged psychological support.

Stress and major cardiovascular events (heart attacks and strokes)

There is a well-established association between psychological stress and heart attacks and strokes, as well as deaths caused by these conditions (Table 6.2). What's more, the relationship between psychological stress and heart disease or stroke has been confirmed by large population studies. Stress contributes to cardiovascular disease not only directly, by triggering the release of adrenaline, but indirectly: distressed people tend to smoke more, to drink excessively, to eat more, and to exercise less.(6)

In a very large INTERHEART study (page 19) on nearly 30 000 patients in 52 countries, stress was one of six major risk factors causing heart attacks. The other five risks were smoking, cholesterol problems, diabetes, hypertension, and abdominal obesity. There were three protective factors: exercise, a high fruit and vegetable diet, and moderate alcohol consumption. Between them, these nine factors

Table 6.2 Stress factors linked to heart attacks

'Stress is a difficult construct, in that no consensus exists with respect to definition or measurement. Further, stress is inevitably a subjective measurement.'
1. Stress at work or home, intermittent (45% increase in risk)
2. Stress at work or home, sustained (117% increase)
3. Financial stress (33% increase)
4. Major life events (48% increase)
5. Depression (55% increase)

Note these are *relative* increases. What really matters is the *absolute risk* of a heart attack, which can be calculated from the Harvard chart (Figs. 3.4 and 3.5), and depends on age, gender, blood pressure, diabetic status, and body mass index. The relative risk from stress increases the absolute risk from the Harvard chart. Source of data and quotation: Rosengren A, et al. Lancet 2004; 364: 953.

(or the lack thereof) explained over 90% of serious heart attacks. So we can see that it is the combination of six adverse factors that provides the background against which heart attacks occur. Each of these factors requires active therapy, and stress is only one of them.

Stress relief and protection of the heart by exercising

The adrenergic system is activated by stress, and increases blood pressure and heart rate. Exercise training stimulates the activity of the anti-stress cholinergic system, which slows the pulse rate at rest and drops the blood pressure. In other words, exercise training protects against the mechanisms triggered by stress. For example, at the start of a heart attack, the adrenergic system is abruptly activated. Experiments performed in my laboratory show that exercise training can protect the heart from the adrenaline-associated damage caused by a sudden blockage of a major coronary artery (Fig. 6.7). This has been confirmed in real life by significant studies showing the protective benefit of exercise training in those who have had heart attacks. Clearly, exercise training is a form of stress relief.

Neurotransmitters: inhibition or stimulation?

Different parts of the brain have different functions, which means that nervous impulses must travel from one part of your brain to another. This is not a simple matter. Although it's easy to see that heart rate and blood pressure are increased by the stimulatory adrenergic system (including both noradrenaline and adrenaline; USA terminology: norepinephrine and epinephrine), the brain is vastly more complex than the heart in structure and function. A huge number of messengers communicate between the many different types of brain cell, and this number varies dramatically from one part of the brain to the next.

As simply as it can be put, the stimulatory system in the brain works via two major systems: (1) the adrenergic messengers of the brain, chief of which is dopamine (closely related to noradrenaline); and (2) serotonin. The dopamine system transmits messages up and down between the front of the brain (the frontal cortex) and sites in the

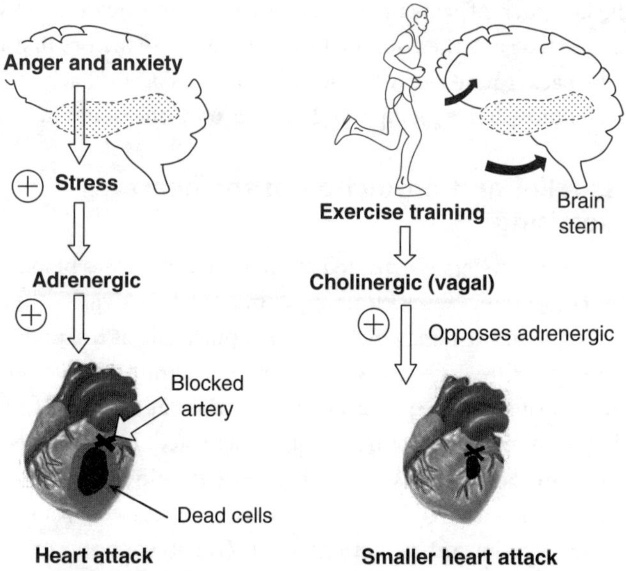

Figure 6.7 Prior exercise training to lessen the stress on the heart. Note the contrasting effect of the alerting adrenergic system, and the activity of the opposing parasympathetic cholinergic system (Table 1.1). Thereby the risk of sudden death in a heart attack is lessened through exercise training. These figures are based on research at the University of Cape Town by Timothy Noakes and Lionel Opie. Modified from Fig. 2 of Grassi G et al. by permission of American Heart Association and Circulation (*Circulation* 1999; 100: 222–225). © Opie.

lower brain, in order to carry out complex functions such as dealing with rewards, pleasure, and euphoria. The serotonin system deals with mood, memory, and cognition, for which it requires more widespread connections, both in the conscious and in the lower brain. Antidepressant drugs act on one or the other of these systems.

Dopamine

Antidepressants that stimulate the dopamine system of the brain enhance mood by increasing the availability of dopamine. They do this by inhibiting the uptake of dopamine back into the nerve ending from where the dopamine was released, so that there is greater stimulation of the next nerve (Fig. 6.8). The end effect is to counter psychological

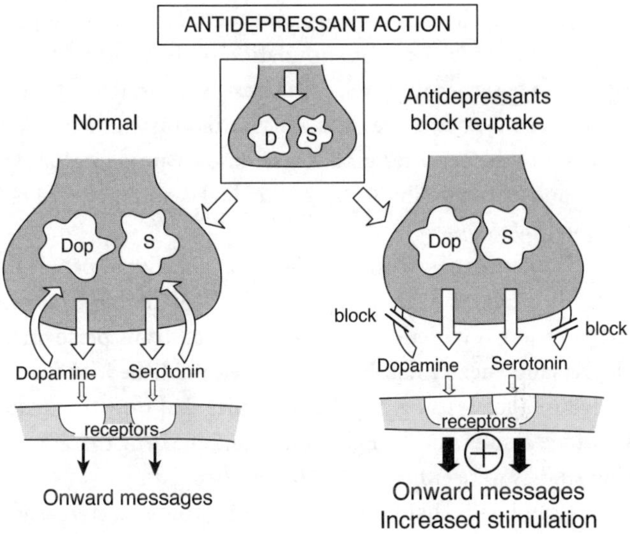

Figure 6.8 Antidepressant drugs and their mechanisms. These agents act at the end of the nerve cells (terminal neurones) where nervous impulses are conducted from one brain cell to the next. An excess amount of each messenger, dopamine (Dop) or serotonin (S), is released, and most of the released messenger is then taken up by the same terminal that released it (reuptake). Antidepressants inhibit the reuptake mechanism, thereby increasing stimulation of the brain. © Opie.

depression, but sometimes at a cost; because dopamine is closely related to noradrenaline, the heart rate may increase and there may be other cardiac side-effects.

In practice, most antidepressants that stimulate the release of dopamine also stimulate the release of serotonin. Conversely, the addictive and dangerous drug cocaine causes intense short-term stimulation of the dopamine system without affecting serotonin levels, giving the pleasurable but transient 'high' typical of this drug.

Serotonin

Other antidepressant drugs act on the serotonin messenger system, which has some functions in common with the dopamine system. Selective serotonin reuptake inhibitors (SSRIs) increase the activity of the serotonin messenger system. This increases neurotransmission and decreases psychological depression, similarly to the dopamine system, yet without any major stimulation of the heart and arteries. Like dopamine, serotonin is released in excess from nerve terminals, and in the normal course of events, most serotonin would be taken up again back into the nerve terminals. Well-known antidepressants such as Prozac and Zoloft inhibit serotonin reuptake, and therefore reduce depression (Fig. 6.8).

However, these drugs may not be nearly as effective as people think. In a recent analysis in the very reliable *New England Journal of Medicine*, it was revealed that of 74 registered trials performed on antidepressants, nearly half had never been published, or they were published in a misleading way. This implies that only those studies with positive results saw the light of day, and the drug therapy results in other studies were either neutral or negative.

The bottom line is that there is no compelling, objective evidence that antidepressants do everything their manufacturers claim they do. Although now incorporated into popular culture, Prozac, Zoloft, and similar drugs should be reserved for major depressive illness, should be prescribed by psychiatrists, and should never be used as a 'pick me up' or to relieve stress. Although uncommon, suicide is now recognized as a serious side-effect of antidepressants, especially in adolescents.

Reward circuits and neuroenhancers

Could it be that another way of reducing stress would be to increase the activity of potentially pleasurable circuits in the brain? Only if we can reach and influence those circuits—and for a long time, we didn't even know where they were.

The frontal cortex, where conscious pleasure and other complex emotions are experienced, is in constant communication with the lower unconscious brain centres, such as those in the mid-brain and brain stem (Fig. 6.9). The brain stem itself is crowded with specialized centres, one of which is the vasomotor centre already discussed. Until very recently, nobody knew that these lower centres participated in forming major conscious goals and emotional drives, for which the technical term is 'goal-directed behaviour'. This means that there are up and down circuits that include the lower brain that

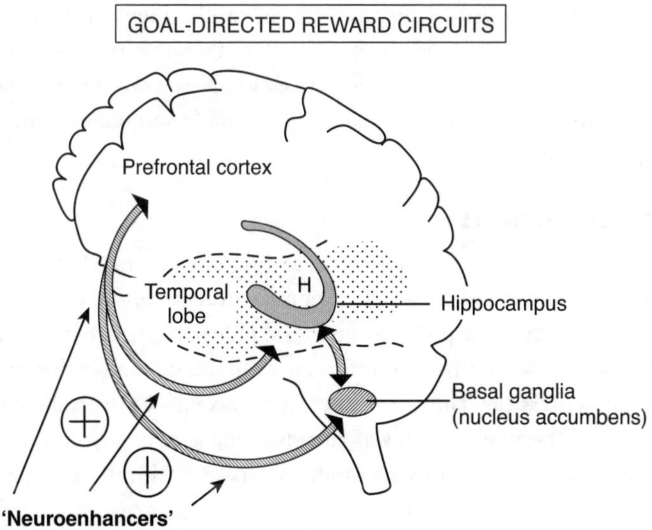

Figure 6.9 Reward circuits. Goal-directed reward-seeking behaviour is not just a function of the conscious cortex of the brain that says 'I will behave in a certain way'; it involves the interaction of signals to and from the mid-brain (hippocampus) and the basal ganglia of the brain stem (technical anatomical term: nucleus accumbens). Such paths are also involved in brain stimulation by 'neuroenhancing' drugs. When reward circuits are repetitively stimulated—for example by nicotine or brain stimulants—the circuits can become entrenched and addictive. (Note that artistic licence has been used here: this drawing does not show the exact situation of the nucleus accumbens, which lies at the top of the brain stem, anatomically much higher than shown here.) © Opie.

are involved in setting life goals, which can then be translated into physical action. These circuits are called reward or reward-related circuits. They travel through a specialized part of the brain stem called the nucleus accumbus.(7)

An example of a person actively stimulating a reward circuit—one that could potentially relieve stress—might be that of the dedicated but relaxed artist. His oil painting begins in the cortex, where the initial urge to paint originates. From there, messages are sent down to the lower brain, only to ascend back up to the cortex to reinforce and develop the creative urge. When repeated often, this 'painter's circuit' could add skill to the painter's art, because the circuit is already there and only needs reinforcement. Further development of the circuit could take place as new ideas come in. But in another type of painter, say someone frenetic like Vincent van Gogh, these same circuits could be used to generate stress even as they stimulate and increase intense artistic output.

Neuroenhancers

A variety of these drugs are now taken by those seeking 'brain gain', especially stressed office and university workers hoping to improve their intellectual output (Figs. 6.9 and 6.10). These are not mood enhancers (at least, that is not their main function), and are not used to treat depression. The oldest of these is Dexedrine (the trade name for dexamfetamine), which was already being used and abused in my student days, followed by its modern derivate Addrall (Table 6.3).

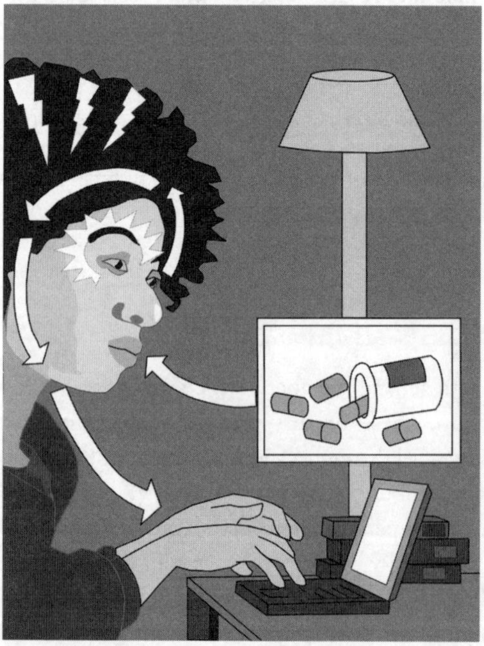

Figure 6.10 Neuroenhancers. A hypothetical university student temporarily sparkling at night under the influence of a neuroenhancer.

Table 6.3 'Neuroenhancers'

1. Dexedrine (dexamfetamine in UK, dextroamphetamine in USA), licensed in UK for refractory Attention Deficit Hyperactivity Disorder; the oldest 'neuroenchancer'
2. Adderall (mixture of amphetamine and dextroamphetamine salts), licensed in USA for Attention Deficit Hyperactivity Disorder
3. Ritalin (methylphenidate), licensed for Attention Deficit Disorder and in USA for narcolepsy; may act in a similar way to Provigil
4. Provigil (modafinil), dopamine stimulator, licensed for excessive daytime sleepiness associated with narcolepsy; also in UK for obstructive sleep apnoea
5. Nootropil (piracetam), may have cholinergic-type mechanism by increased levels of the neurotransmitter acetylcholine; licensed in UK but not USA for myoclonus, a type of muscular spasm; licensed in South Africa for 'involution problems related to ageing', which could mean anything.

Cautions: None of these are licensed to increase brain activity nor as a 'neuroenhancer'. Dexedrine, Adderall, Ritalin, and Provigil are agents that stimulate the adrenergic system. As a group, they may increase heart rate and blood pressure. They are not suited for use in middle-aged or elderly persons at risk of hypertension or heart problems.

Ritalin (methylphenidate) and Provigil (modafinil) stimulate the dopamine system of the brain. Nootropil (piracetam) acts differently—by stimulating another neurotransmitter, acetylcholine. Increasingly, stressed intellectual workers around the globe, especially aspirant American academics, are now using these agents. Often, they carefully dilute the dose to get stimulation of the brain without side-effects, such as increased heart rate and blood pressure. Neuroenhancers taken judiciously usually don't leave serious side-effects behind, but in some they become addictive or precipitate serious psychiatric conditions.

A reliable current study from the National Institute on Drug Abuse in the USA, using ultra-modern brain imaging techniques, showed that modafinil increased the dopamine content of the human brain, including that of the nucleus accumbens.(8) This means it acts on the reward circuits (Fig. 6.9), the reward in this case being greater mental stimulation, but because it involves the nucleus accumbens, repeated use can result in addiction. Over-stimulation may also have a rebound negative effect.

Mind over matter?

Let's go back to exercise. Similar circuits may interact up and down between the cortex and lower centres to explain the 'central governor' hypothesis in greater detail; in other words, the possibility that a central control mechanism can extend the physical limits of exercise (Fig. 6.3). It seems 'mind over matter' may partly be the simple act of positively enhancing existing reward circuits. Conversely, similar circuits can be stimulated by stress-generated thoughts and emotional bodily reactions, leading to a fear that builds up as the circuits repeat themselves. Thus 'negative reward' circuits can also be generated. In the case of drugs such as nicotine and the neuroenhancers, an initially positive reward can become powerfully self-enhancing, and strong enough to imprison the person in addictive patterns—with major negative effects on the health of the heart.

Summary

The mind can have a powerful influence over the body, and in particular over the heart and cardiovascular system. Feats of extreme physical endurance show us that a trained body and motivated mind have the capacity to extend physical limits. It is likely that we have a central command system, which probably works through interaction between conscious higher and unconscious lower brain centres.

The emotions also play an important role in several types of heart disease. Psychological stress can increase adrenergic stimulation via the messengers (adrenaline and noradrenaline, also called epinephrine and norepinephrine), which may cause or aggravate cardiovascular diseases such as hypertension and coronary artery disease. Extreme examples are those unfortunate individuals who drop dead during an earthquake, or die suddenly from a stress-related stroke.

Although some people reduce stress through psychotherapy, the best measures against stress-promoted diseases (such as hypertension and heart attacks) are strict control of blood pressure by taking the correct medication, exercising regularly, lowering cholesterol through diet and drugs, achieving a normal weight, and definitely no smoking. Exercise training stimulates the activity of the parasympathetic cholinergic nervous system (Table 1.1), which slows the pulse rate at rest and drops the blood pressure—these protective effects are opposite to the adverse effects of over-stimulation of the adverse adrenergic system.

These measures help to protect the heart from the overstimulation often caused by stress. Protection of the brain is much more complex and the subject of intense investigation. Life-style measures, high dose of omega-3 fatty acids, and treatment of cardiovascular disease provide the background. To counter brain shrinkage in the elderly, novel new data albeit in a small study argue for high doses of vitamins B12, B6, and folic acid (page 154). Note my reservation about high dose folic acid in those with heart disease.

Depression is in some ways the opposite of stress, and so one therapeutic strategy is to simulate stress by using antidepressant drugs that increase the levels of stimulating messengers in the brain—at the risk of various side-effects. Goal-directed reward-seeking behaviour can be explained by an interaction between the thinking brain (cortex), the middle brain, and the lower brain. These 'reward' circuits can be consciously triggered and frequently repeated to become self-perpetuating circuits, which explains the strong habit patterns that form—which may either exaggerate or reduce levels of stress. Drugs called neuroenhancers induce brain stimulation artificially by acting on these circuits, but users face the potential danger of addiction.

Chapter 7

Cognitive Function and Memory Loss

Lionel Opie and Joseph Raimondo

What is cognition? The word is taken from the Latin 'cognitio', meaning the process of acquiring knowledge, along with study, recognition, social connectivity, and discovery (Fig. 7.1). Cognition implies perceiving and thinking and being aware and responsive to the world around us. To help understand the term we need to go back nearly 400 years to René Descartes, who in 1619 made the immortal statement 'I think, therefore I am' (*Cogito, ergo sum*). He then expanded: 'I know plainly that I can achieve an easier and more evident perception of my own mind than of anything else.' Cognition is just that—the ability to perceive one's own mind.

As human lifespan becomes longer and longer, it becomes increasingly important to maintain a clear mind and a functioning memory system. Normal ageing causes a certain inevitable rate of decline of memory. But often in middle age, memory seems to be slipping faster than it should. Memory is clearly one of the most important functions of the brain, and memory loss is probably the aspect of cognitive function that most directly concerns most ageing people. Suppose that you, as the reader, are doubting your memory, how should you approach this problem? We will try to answer this later in the chapter, although there are no magic solutions.

This chapter will focus on preserving memory as one of the most important elements of cognition. We will be covering the molecular mechanisms of memory, diseases that impair it (including the dreaded Alzheimer's), steps to preserve memory (Table 7.1), and the numerous dietary changes and supplements that may (or may not) help to combat age-related memory loss.

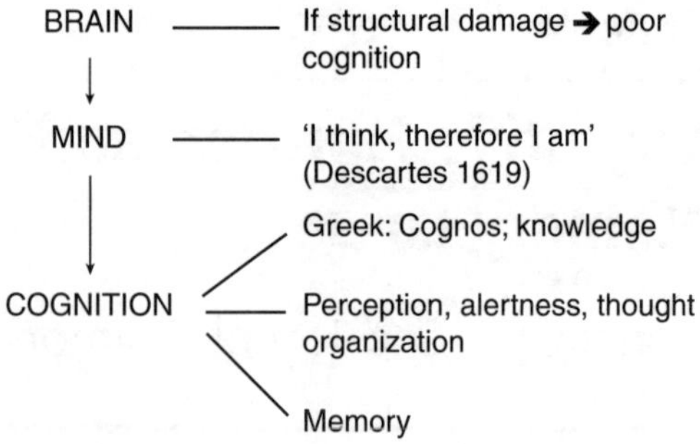

Figure 7.1 Cognition is a quality that encompasses memory. Cognition requires a functioning brain and mind.

Table 7.1 Memory preservation or possible enhancement

Create a stronger input of memory signals
Look and listen carefully
Repeat silently what you hear and want to remember
Concentrate intensely; shut out external events
Enhance the emotional significance of the input
Mental training
Lifestyle changes, for long-term protection and benefit
Regular physical exercise
Avoid obesity and minimize risk of diabetes
Avoid excess alcohol
Mediterranean food pattern; note high omega-3 fatty acids
In elderly, high dose vitamins B12 and B6. Add folic acid if no heart disease
Avoid arterial disease: no smoking, control cholesterol, blood pressure
In older adults: exclude atrial fibrillation (check pulse rate)
Psychotropic drugs
Only under medical guidance
Drugs that you can try (no guarantees)
Aspirin
Ibuprofen (Brufen)
Viagra

Alzheimer's disease is the best known and major cause of serious memory impairment. First described by the German brain specialist of that name about a century ago, it remains a disease that is not well understood. Here the memory loss is major and socially disabling – for example, parking a car when shopping and then having absolutely no idea what had happened to it (as happened to one of our friends). In reality, anyone able to buy this book is very unlikely to have established Alzheimer's disease, although cognitive loss looms for almost everyone as the years go by. The burning question is: how severe will the loss be?

Definitions of cognitive loss and memory

Cognitive loss extends beyond a simple decrease in memory to embrace a wider set of mental deficits. These affect the way we interact with the world around us. For instance, tests of cognitive function probe a wide variety of skills, including orientation in space, attention, drawing diagrams, performing simple arithmetic, and spelling words backwards. Ideally cognitive tests would also assess more nebulous qualities such as creative thought and social interaction. Note that cognition excludes emotional reactions or expressions.

In practice, cognitive impairment can readily and roughly be estimated by a simplified test called the mini-mental state examination (MMSE), a brief 30-point questionnaire that only takes about ten minutes to complete. This test is also used to monitor changes in cognitive impairment over time, so it is an effective way to monitor someone's decline with age or their response to treatment.

The most crucial components of our cognitive life are the ability to learn and to remember new information. During the ageing process, the defect varies in magnitude from 'moderately inconvenient benign forgetfulness to devastating losses associated with Alzheimer's disease and certain ischemic episodes'(1).

It is memory that we are generally most worried about, because memory is so dependent on self-assessment and so essential for everyday function. Here we suggest a guide to self-management (Fig. 7.2). Technically, there are two types of memory—first, 'knowing what is what', which means recalling events of the past or general knowledge, as opposed to 'know how to do it' memory, which includes learning

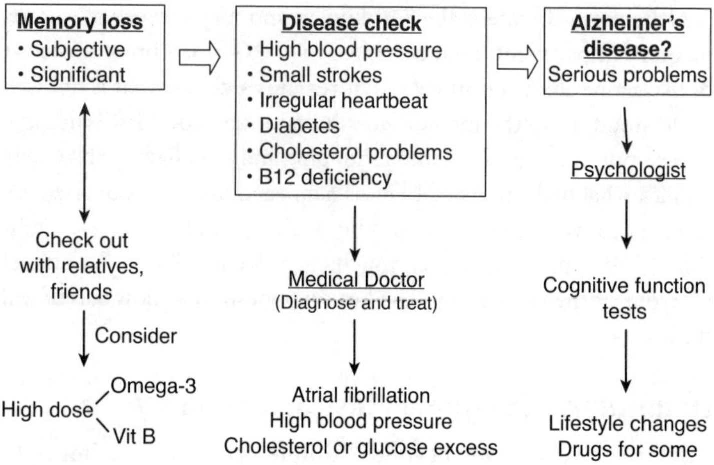

Figure 7.2 A reader's guide to self-management of suspected memory loss. Vit=Vitamin. © Opie.

actions and skills such as riding a bicycle.[2] It is the 'knowing what is what' that we usually mean when we think of memory in everyday use.

The mechanisms of memory

We all know what it feels like not to be able to remember something important, the way it 'slips the mind'. What we don't know is exactly how memory works. It's helpful if we understand that memory can be divided into short- and long-term components. Short-term memory is like typing a sentence into your word processor. The sentence remains in the computer's temporary storage ('memory'), but if a power failure shuts down the computer or you close the file without first saving it to the hard drive, the sentence will be lost. Saving the sentence means transferring the information from temporary storage to long-term storage on the hard drive, in the form of a file that can be retrieved later. People with good memories can 'press the correct buttons' in the brain and call up information easily, while those with poor memories need time to remember, or seem prone to forget altogether, apparently forever.

So memory resembles material saved onto a computer drive awaiting recall. Sometimes a memory sticks, other times it doesn't, depending in part on whatever else is influencing the brain at that time. As we know, some experiences are more easily remembered than others. Emotional context can massively enhance memory storage. Which do you remember better, your first kiss or your first bank statement?

Loss of memory and the hippocampus

Many parts of the brain are implicated in memory. Some of the most important areas lie deep within the temporal lobes. These lobes are situated on either side of the brain, roughly beneath the temple bones on either side of the skull. Lying inside the temporal lobe is a part of the brain called the hippocampus. Its name is the Latin word for seahorse, due to its rather curious shape. If one brain area could be thought of as the 'memory centre', the hippocampus would be it (Fig. 7.3). Another important region of the temporal lobe is the temporal cortex, the outer superficial layer.

To better understand the role these parts of the brain play in memory, we must look at clinical observations of patients with damage to these particular areas. The most famous patient in the history of brain science was a man known as HM. In a desperate attempt to treat severe epilepsy, both his temporal lobes, which include the hippocampus, were

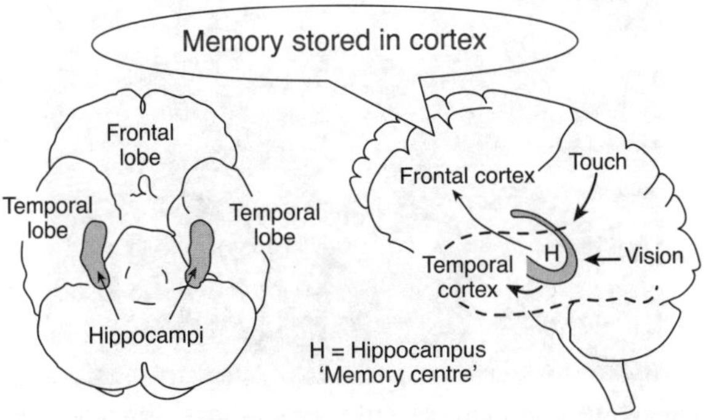

Figure 7.3 Memory map. Information about our experiences of the world around us is first picked up by the sensory organs (such as the eyes and ears). Signals from these organs are processed by sensory areas in the brain before being sent to the hippocampus (H). The hippocampus, or 'memory centre', then converts these 'memory triggers' into long-term memories to be stored in the cortex. © Opie.

surgically removed. Although his epilepsy was cured, he was left with profound memory impairment. His short-term memory was intact, and he could remember his childhood in exquisite detail, but after his surgery he was unable to commit any new events to long-term memory. For the next fifty-five years, each time he met a friend, ate a meal, or walked in the woods, it was as if for the first time.

Another patient suffered from serious damage to the hippocampus (Fig. 7.4) as a result of a viral infection of the brain at age 40. The result was similar: severe loss of memory for recent events, even though he could recall exact details of the area where he grew up.

From these and from many other patients we have learned that the hippocampus plays a critical role in the formation of new memories. As Fig. 7.3 demonstrates, information about our experiences in the outside world originally stem from the senses (eyes, ears, and to

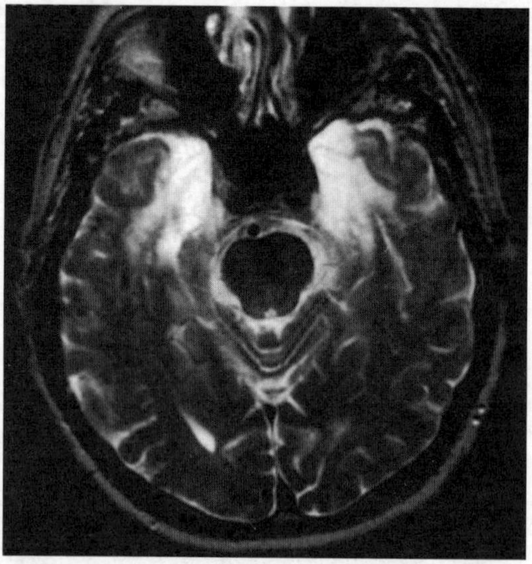

Figure 7.4 White brain and recent memory loss. This radiological view of the brain from above shows in white the hippocampus after damage by a viral infection. The result was a complete inability to form any new long-term memories. Reproduced from Teng E and Squire LR. Memory for places learned long ago is intact after hippocampal damage. *Nature* 1999; 400: 675–7, by permission of Macmillan Publishers Ltd.

a lesser extent touch, smell, and taste). Signals from these sensory organs are processed by sensory areas in the brain before being sent to the hippocampus. The hippocampus then converts these 'memory triggers' into long-term memories to be stored in the outer, cortical parts of the brain .

Stimulating the cortex of the temporal lobe

A famous Canadian neurosurgeon, Dr Wilder Penfield, regularly opened up brains of patients by cutting a flap in the bony skull, all under local anaesthesia. That is, his patients were kept fully conscious during his operations. He then electrically stimulated the exposed cortex (remember the cortex is the superficial outer layer of the brain) with a pointed electrode. He was trying to find the exact origin of a certain type of epilepsy that originated in the temporal lobe. His theory was that he could then excise that part of the cortex that caused the epilepsy. In fact, he unexpectedly found that by this method of stimulation of the temporal cortex, he evoked complex memories from the distant past in his patients, memories that they had apparently totally forgotten. This shows that the superficial layer of the temporal lobe, the cortex, forms part of the brain's 'memory store'.

Taken together, these studies show that the hippocampus, located in the deeper parts of the temporal lobe, is required for acquisition of memories, which are then transferred to widespread cortical areas for long-term storage. These areas include the temporal cortex and the frontal cortex. Many different parts of the brain are thus involved in the memory process.

Memory messengers

How are memories stored in the brain? Memories are not held within a single brain cell (one memory per cell). If this were the case, every time a brain cell died, its accompanying memory would be lost forever. Fortunately, the brain employs a more robust form of memory storage. A memory is stored as a complex pattern of connections between an interactive group of many brain cells distributed in a particular area. These groups of cells are linked by the patterns of electrical and chemical activity that connect the cells. The technical term for such activity is electrochemical, because it is partly electrical, which explains the very rapid conduction of electrical impulses along the length of a brain cell. Another part is chemical, which refers to the release of chemicals from the ending of one brain cell. These travel across an infinitesimally small space, called the synapse, between one cell and the next (Fig. 7.5). The number of cells in the brain is beyond comprehension, and can only be estimated at something like one hundred billion (10^{11}), with about one hundred trillion synapses (10^{14}).

Memory formation

First, an event recorded by the eyes or ears must reach the memory storage sites in the brain. The signals that represent information about the world around us (flashes of light, loud noises, sharp smells, and so on) must travel from the sense organs (eyes and ears) to parts of the brain able to interpret this information. Each sense has its own area in the brain. For instance, the visual area has circuits of brain cells that might decide that the flashes of light represent a chicken crossing the road. This information about the chicken and its pedestrian habits is then sent to the hippocampus and other memory areas for eventual storage as a long-term memory in the cortex.

Communication between brain cells

To successfully carry out this sort of information processing, brain cells must be able to send each other signals over long distances. Brain cells or neurones differ from most other cells in the body by having very prolonged wire-like extensions of two types, called either axons or dendrites (Fig. 7.5). These resemble tendrils, or even the arms of an octopus (except that the body of an octopus only has eight branches whereas there are many more dendrites in brain cells). Dendrites receive signals from other brain cells—they are the 'input' wires to the brain cells. Each brain cell has many dendrites branching out profusely, becoming thinner with each branch until these minute branches terminate, forming a tree-like structure. Whereas each brain cell has very many dendrites, each has only one axon. Axons send signals to other brain cells; they are the 'output' wires of a cell. The axon of a

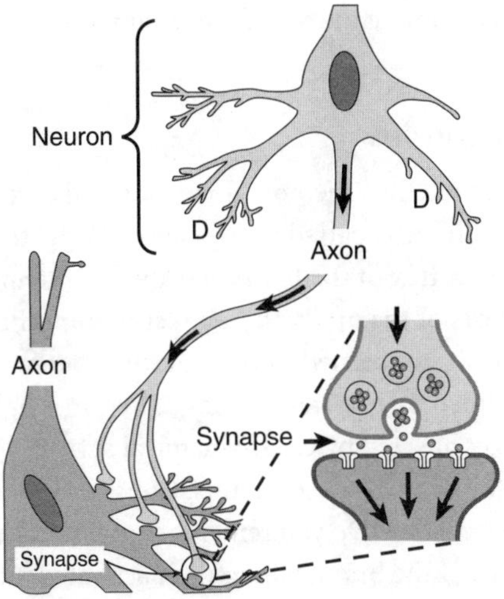

Figure 7.5 How signals travel between brain cells. This is a simplified diagram of communication between brain cells or neurones (neurone is the Greek word for nerve). Incoming signals from other brain cells arrive at the dendrites (D), which branch out like feelers from the main body of the brain cells to pick up incoming messages. These then travel as ultra-rapid electrical impulses down the much longer axon. When the impulses reach a connection point with another cell, something like an intersection, chemical messengers called neurotransmitters (such as acetylcholine and glutamate) are released. These jump across the very narrow gap between cells known as the synapse (from the Greek, to join) as shown in the insert and in Fig. 7.6. The neurotransmitters then activate receptors on the dendrites of the receiving cell to generate a new electrical impulse and send it along to the next cell and so forth, keeping the signal going. © Opie & Raimondo.

brain cell connects with the dendrites of the next cell at specialized junctions or gaps called synapses (Fig. 7.5).

When an electrical signal travelling down an axon reaches a synapse, it causes chemical messengers (called neurotransmitters) to be released. These move across the synapse to bind to specialized receptors on one of the dendrites of the next cell. These receptors in turn generate another electrical impulse that continues the propagation of the signal (Fig. 7.5). By controlling the strength of connections between brain cells, synapses are critically involved in the process of forming and maintaining the specific signalling patterns that make up a memory.

Recall of memories

Less well understood than memory formation is the exact mechanism of memory recall, also called retrieval. As long-term memories are stored in the cortex of the brain, mostly in the temporal lobe but also in other lobes of the brain, there must be a mechanism that sets the circuit of cells concerned with the stored memory in motion. As already outlined, memories are not stored in single cells, but in circuits of cells connected by electrochemical activity. Accessing such memories must reactivate these circuits. Conscious memory recall, in response to the question 'Do you remember ...?' starts in the cortex of the frontal lobes of the brain, which then activates the memory circuits predominantly in the temporal cortex.[3] Delayed recall, the common 'it's on the tip of my tongue' experience, suggests that activating the correct memory circuit can be subject to delay. By letting the mind wander, we are sometimes able to activate part of a memory circuit serendipitously, often triggering an entire storage circuit to become active, thereby causing a flood of sudden recall.

Neurotransmitters

Neurotransmitters are the chemical messengers that carry a signal across the synapse between brain cells. Two specific neurotransmitters, acetylcholine and glutamate[3], are particularly involved in learning and memory formation. Generally, each brain cell releases only one type of neurotransmitter.

Acetylcholine

This is the same compound that mediates the effects of natural sleep by slowing the heart rate. It is also the compound that is increased by regular exercise training, which in turn promotes memory. In the brain, acetylcholine is extremely important for memory formation. Brain cells that release acetylcholine are exceptional in that they branch extensively, creating synapses (Fig. 7.5) with a very large number of other cells. This enables these specialized brain cells to influence the general level of activity within entire brain areas. We do not know exactly how acetylcholine contributes to memory formation. However, we do know that in Alzheimer's disease, there is a loss of acetylcholine-producing cells, especially in the temporal lobes. In addition, blocking acetylcholine receptors with drugs impairs memory formation. Conversely, drugs that act in a similar way to acetylcholine (cholinergic drugs) have been shown to improve memory. These are now being used in the treatment of Alzheimer's disease.

Glutamate

Unlike acetylcholine-releasing cells, brain cells that release glutamate connect only to a small number of other cells in very specific circuits (chains of connected cells). The activity within such a circuit might represent a particular memory. The strength of the connection between two cells in a circuit is not fixed, but can be strengthened or weakened, a process known as synaptic plasticity. Receptors for glutamate play an important role in this process, and are therefore integral to memory formation. In Alzheimer's disease, glutamate receptors appear to malfunction; new drugs being developed to treat this disease aim to target these receptors.

Plasticity and long-term potentiation

Memories are stored as patterns of connections across many brain cells. Therefore, to form a new memory, the brain must be able to change the strength of connections between cells. This may happen in several different ways. Firstly, a brain cell can release more neurotransmitter every time an electrical signal sent along its axon reaches the synapse. Secondly, the brain cell receiving the signal can become more sensitive to the neurotransmitter released by synthesizing more receptors (Fig. 7.6). All these processes serve to help and strengthen the future transmission of a signal across the synapse.

The lasting strengthening of connections between two brain cells is called long-term potentiation (LTP). LTP is thought to be one of the primary cellular mechanisms important for long-term memory formation. It results from repeated, strong signals being sent across the synapse. This triggers the two brain cells involved to strengthen their connection in the ways mentioned above. Plasticity processes

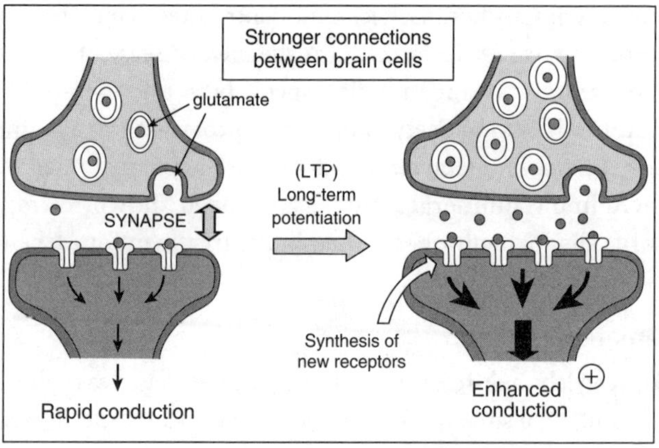

Figure 7.6 Strengthening the basis of memory: enhanced conduction between brain cells. On the left, messenger molecules or neurotransmitters such as glutamate are released at the endings of brain cells. Crossing the synapse, the gap between cells, they pass on the signal so that information is rapidly transmitted from one cell to the next to make a memory circuit. On the right, memory can be enhanced if an increased number of glutamate molecules interact with more receptors to promote conduction of the impulse across the synapse, making it faster and stronger. This requires the synthesis of new proteins, technically called long-term potentiation (LTP, see text). Such strengthening of connections between brain cells is the basis of the formation of a new memory. Of course, if we knew how to make more of these memory-facilitating proteins, we might well be able to revolutionize the treatment of age-related memory loss. In true Alzheimer's disease, the abnormal beta-amyloid peptide is believed to block the receptors for the neurotransmitter glutamate, thereby impairing memory formation.[4,5]

such as LTP are known to be impaired in Alzheimer's, possibly explaining the very prominent memory problems that are a feature of this disease.

Causes of memory loss

Whatever memory is, it commonly deteriorates with advancing age. Part of this deterioration is often ascribed to the fact that as we age, the number of our brain cells falls because these cells cannot duplicate themselves. However, we now know that this is not entirely true.

Controversial and recent research suggests that at least in some circumstances, the situation is much like that in the heart. Here, cells do not usually duplicate, but in exceptional circumstances, such as in response to a heart attack, even mature heart cells can divide to help 'rescue' the organ. Likewise, new brain cells can exceptionally be generated in the adult brain. Nonetheless, ageing remains the most common cause of memory loss, followed by strokes, and only then by Alzheimer's disease.

Just as in the case of the ageing heart, various aspects of cerebral function in the brain slowly deteriorate with age. The volume of the living brain can be measured using the technique of magnetic resonance imaging (MRI), and this clearly shows us that the volume of the brain declines with age. There is shrinkage (atrophy), especially in the posterior regions, as well as in all the frontal sites. Besides the loss of brain substance, the brain that remains may undergo degenerative changes. However, the quantity of grey matter that lies just beneath the outer layer of the brain, where the cell bodies of brain cells reside, reassuringly remains about the same. The real problem is that the white matter that contains the connecting 'wires' between brain cells shrinks. This means that over time, brain circuits become less well connected 'with their neighbours and friends.'[(6)] Loss of connectivity means loss of circuits that sustain memory.

It would be wonderful if modern medicine could aid us in recovering 'lost memories' as we grow older. Unfortunately, this remains a pipe-dream. More realistic action, to be considered later in this chapter, would be to take preventative action to retain those memories we already possess.

Strokes, high blood pressure, and memory loss

Strokes result when a diseased artery either ruptures to let blood plough into the brain tissue, or blocks up to deprive the brain of its life-giving oxygen and nourishment (Fig. 7.7). When there is a series of strokes, typically some small and some large, then the end result can be serious loss of brain function (dementia) caused by multiple areas of brain cell death, technically called infarction (which means stuffed-in dead cells). Besides loss of memory, there may be other

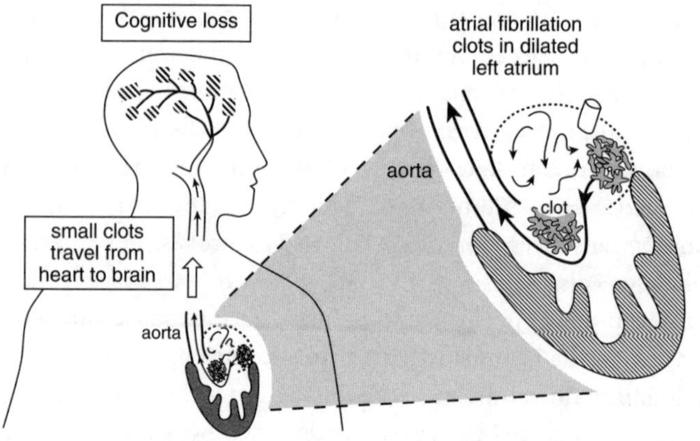

Figure 7.7 Small strokes can block memory. Stroke results either when a diseased artery ruptures to let blood burst into the brain tissue, or when the artery gets blocked up, depriving the brain of life-giving oxygen and nourishment. Note the possible cardiac causes of clots travelling to the brain (see also Fig. 2.2). © Opie.

personality changes such as severe depression or agitation. After each stroke, whether small enough to be silent or serious enough to be obvious, cognitive loss and memory decline accelerate. The major cause of stroke is vascular disease, of which high blood pressure is a prime cause, with high blood cholesterol and diabetes being other major causes, exactly as in the case of coronary heart disease. These factors may combine to promote disease in the large carotid arteries that convey most of the blood to the brain (Fig. 7.7).

Each of the major factors promoting arterial disease (abnormal blood pressure, cholesterol, and high blood glucose) can be controlled by modern drugs and can be prevented at least in part by lifestyle changes. Of these three, diagnosis and management of blood pressure is most important, followed by care of blood glucose and diabetes, and finally control of cholesterol levels. All these will be considered in greater detail later in this chapter.

Small strokes, cerebral white matter, and memory

The advent of magnetic resonance imaging (MRI), a new technology that allows doctors to image the brain, has helped to define the physical basis for the loss of memory in small strokes that are otherwise clinically silent. In repetitive small strokes, degeneration of the brain is associated with damage to what is known as white matter. White matter is comprised of dense bundles of axons. Its destruction destroys the connections between brain cells, including those involved in memory, thereby destroying the memory itself. These abnormalities are associated with but not specific to hypertension and memory loss. For instance, an example of white matter destruction due to a viral disease is shown in Fig. 7.4.

How do these lesions arise? The blood supply to white matter is very specialized. The penetrating arteries come from the network of larger arteries located on the surface of the brain. These penetrating arteries run at right angles to the surface for about 20–50 mm until the artery ends abruptly. In technical terms, that means that there are very few links, called anastomoses, between these blood vessels. Thus, the blood supply to the white matter becomes seriously threatened and potentially inadequate when there is any episodic fall in the blood pressure or when the arterial wall is damaged by hypertension, high blood cholesterol, diabetes, or age. All these factors impact adversely on these small penetrating arteries. Not surprisingly, problems of the penetrating arteries are also more common in those who have had big strokes, or in those with Alzheimer's disease.

High blood pressure and memory loss

Of all the adverse influences on white matter, that with the clearest correlation to memory loss is high blood pressure, probably because it directly damages blood vessels. The greater the blood pressure, the greater the severity of the white matter lesions and the degree of memory loss. These studies strongly suggest that high blood pressure causes or else promotes the development of white matter lesions. Thus common sense would say: look for and treat high blood pressure. High blood pressure is linked to memory loss, the evidence being that: (1) those with high blood pressure as a group have impaired cognitive capacity; and (2) there are physical changes found in the brain of hypertensives. These changes include increased brain shrinkage[(7)], abnormal white matter (as in Fig. 7.4), and decreased blood flow to the temporal lobes of the brain.

Alzheimer's disease

Besides ageing and strokes, the other main cause of memory loss is Alzheimer's disease. When fully developed, as first described in a patient only in her 50s by Alzheimer in Germany just over 100 years ago, it is a somewhat uncommon condition in which loss of memory and cognitive function are sufficiently serious to severely limit normal social exchange and activity. However, in its more incipient forms, Alzheimer's disease begins as mild but progressive loss of memory (cognitive decline). This is much more common. Diagnosis is made by psychiatrists with the aid of tests of memory function, brain scans such as those showing defects in glucose uptake by the Alzheimer's brain,(7) or more commonly by the demonstration of shrinkage of relevant parts of the brain on an MRI (magnetic resonance imaging) scan.

Plaques and tangles

In an advanced case, samples of tissue from the brain show two characteristic abnormalities. These are typical solid-looking plaques of congealed protein (technically called amyloid-beta peptide plaques) and secondly, the formation of thick tangled fibres within brain cells. The result is that some areas resemble puddles of accumulated sludge, whereas the nerve cells begin to look as if they have exploded and turned into messy tangles of string.(6) Typically these changes occur in that part of the brain that mediates memory, namely the temporal lobes. Of these typical changes, the amyloid plaques can be imaged using very sophisticated and not generally available brain scanning techniques.(8)

Not enough is known about the causation of these plaques and fibrillary changes to take specific preventative steps, even though we know that such lesions can in turn block nourishment of brain cells and promote cell death. Furthermore, the plaques can induce a local inflammatory response that in turn accelerates plaque formation. The opposing argument, supported by a recent negative therapeutic trial, is that amyloid plaques are merely an epiphenomenon of an underlying defect in some other pathological process that is the real cause of memory loss.(9)

From loss of memory to Alzheimer's

Another unsolved problem is whether Alzheimer's disease is a unique and clearly defined entity, or whether it blends with exaggerated forms of other causes of severe mental impairment such as age-related mental deterioration or advanced vascular disease. Both types of brain cell abnormality found in Alzheimer's disease (amyloid plaques and tangles) can occur with ageing.[10] Thus the normal modest memory loss of ageing could become severe enough (the pre-Alzheimer stage) to blend into Alzheimer's disease. This controversial concept of a gradient of progression from age-related memory loss to Alzheimer's disease raises the issue of how to recognize the very common early stages and, if possible, to arrest further deterioration into the full-blown disease. It also follows that significant memory loss should be actively investigated (Fig. 7.2) and treated as early as possible.

Differences between Alzheimer's disease and normal ageing. Brain shrinkage.

Much information comes from a large and very prolonged population study, OPTIMA (Oxford Project to Investigate Memory and Ageing), started 22 years ago.[11] The first major finding in 1994 was that the medial temporal lobe had the greatest concentration of characteristic neurofibrillary tangles and that this part of the brain shrank about ten times more rapidly in those with Alzheimer's disease than in normal ageing. This could not just be an acceleration of normal ageing, but rather was a disease in its own right and the result of 'some catastrophic event in the brain'. Thus these experts argue that Alzheimer's is a disease in its own right, and not just the extreme form of age-related memory loss.

Despite being a specific disease, the origin of Alzheimer's has a multiplicity of causes according to the Oxford group. This concept of a specific disease caused by multiple interactive factors is similar to that of coronary artery disease, a very specific entity with many factors contributing to it, including genes, age, and cholesterol. Thus Alzheimer's is a slowly developing disease caused by multiple predisposing factors, some potentially modifiable, occurring on top of a particular genetic makeup. Current Oxford studies on elderly persons with mild cognitive loss, show that high dose vitamins B12, B6 and folic acid counter brain shrinkage, an early Alzheimer change.[12]

Gene changes

There is a gene that is strongly related to the relatively early but also uncommon onset of Alzheimer's disease in middle age, as described in Alzheimer's original patient. This is the gene for apolipoprotein E4. It is modestly associated with increased vascular disease, but strongly with inherited Alzheimer's. Does measuring this gene help to determine which sufferers of mild memory loss are at higher risk of genuine Alzheimer's disease? The answer is yes but only if the gene is fully expressed (homozygous), which only occurred in about 4% of those tested in one research trial.(13) Presumably similar genetic information could be obtained by checking the family history for Alzheimer's disease.

Steps to maintain memory: measures that should work

Treatment of blood pressure

Because of the clear relationship between hypertension, memory impairment, and white matter lesions, it is most important to treat hypertension vigorously, with one of the target end-points being reduction of memory loss. Memory loss can be a step on the way to serious mental impairment (dementia); it is therefore not surprising that treatment of systolic (top value) hypertension in the elderly reduces the incidence of dementia by half. The bottom line is that if 1000 patients with hypertension were treated with antihypertensive drugs for five years, 19 cases of dementia would be prevented. The evidence that treatment of high blood pressure reduces stroke is extremely strong. Reduction of overt stroke is logically associated with reduction of minor strokes with better maintenance of memory and cognitive function.

Which blood pressures are desirable?

The limits of normality are clear, being below 140/90 mmHg on repetitive values carefully taken. Currently, the ideal blood pressure (BP) is regarded as about 115/75 mmHg, and higher values merge into the pre-hypertensive values above 130/80 mmHg but below 140/90 mmHg (Table 2.1). In the pre-hypertensive group, meaning those that are likely to develop full-blown hypertension with time, the suboptimal BP should be treated by lifestyle measures. It is likely, but not yet fully established, that any antihypertensive drug dropping the systolic (higher) pressure would protect cognitive function and memory. Some drugs such as those blocking the effects of angiotensin (the arterial constrictor) may do this better than others. Thus, the simple message is that higher pressures must come down below 140 mmHg and ideally below 130 mmHg. Don't forget that although you may feel very well you may still have high blood pressure that can harm your memory. Some even call hypertension the silent killer. Remedy? Get your blood pressure measured.

When should treatment be started?

Of special interest is the association of memory loss and abnormal white matter lesions with hypertension in the middle aged. Such formation of white matter lesions starts in middle age, not just in the older ages, so that the sooner blood pressure lowering treatment is started, the better. Common sense and expert opinion (but not properly controlled studies) propose that blood pressure reduction by any mode, including exercise training, weight loss, salt reduction, and drug therapy would reduce major and minor strokes and hence help to maintain memory. While much more needs to be learned, it is clear that high blood pressure predisposes to stroke, that stroke predisposes to memory impairment, and that prevention of stroke helps to maintain memory. Measures that limit large strokes should also limit small memory-impairing strokes. Blood pressure control should begin in early mid-life, because an increase in blood pressure at that time can be followed by a later-life cognitive decline.

Treatment of arterial disease to preserve memory

Back to cholesterol to explain memory defects?

Experimentally, the favourite animal model of Alzheimer's disease is a genetically modified mouse with a pattern of memory defects similar to those associated with the inherited type of human Alzheimer's disease. However, the genetic mutation is not essential. Recent intriguing studies show that normal mice given a high-fat and high-cholesterol diet can develop Alzheimer's disease with typical beta plaques, thereby focusing on the role of cholesterol. The explanation could be that cholesterol is required for the synthesis of beta-amyloid. This does not mean that drugs controlling blood cholesterol such as a powerful group called the statins will necessarily help to prevent or to treat Alzheimer's disease, though there are some positive preliminary studies, both in experimental animals and in patients.

Can statins help?

Four retrospective observational studies have linked statin use to decreased development of Alzheimer's disease. If this association were true, it still would not be clear whether the mechanism is protection of blood vessels as a result of lipid-lowering or a specific statin effect on the amyloid plaques. The limited benefits from statins such as atorvastatin (Lipitor), simvastatin (now over the counter in the United Kingdom), and many others show the need for bigger and longer trials to be performed in order to confirm these effects.

Exercising the body and weight loss to improve memory

Exercise can jog the mind. 'Be smart, exercise your heart.'(14) Several major studies link increased physical exercise to decreased dementia,(15) that is, improved or better-preserved cognitive skills. Looking at older adults, a Boston-based study found that higher levels of physical activity, which is not the same as exercise training, were linked especially to greater executive function—that is the ability to translate commands into action such as drawing a clock to show a certain time.(16) Other studies show that aerobic fitness is associated with reduced age-induced loss of brain tissue in the hippocampus, the part of the brain that is essential to memory.(17)

Experimentally, exercise increases brain growth factors in the hippocampus, and counters the adverse effects of a high fat, high sugar diet on these growth factors.(18,19)

Physical training and memory

Many observational studies show that physical activity delays cognitive decline, which means better memory, but thus far there are only two randomized trials of note. Firstly, in adults with subjective self-diagnosed loss of memory and thus at risk of Alzheimer's disease, a carefully designed and monitored study on 138 people of mean age 69 years showed that six months of organized exercise training modestly improved cognition.[20] In another prospective and well-designed study, exercise training improved cognitive function over 12 months in women aged 65–75 years.[21]

Exercise and endorphins

What are endorphins and how do they relate to memory? Strenuous exercise releases endorphins from the base of the brain where these complex opium-like compounds are made. This explains why those who exercise strenuously 'feel good'. From the evolutionary point of view, why should endorphins have evolved in response to strenuous running? The endorphin system may have protected early humans either when fleeing from danger or allowed them to chase wild animals whilst hunting for longer. This proposed evolutionary concept would explain why the type of exercise that evokes endorphins must be aerobic—resistance exercise (like picking up weights) has no effect on endorphin release.[22]

But what do endorphins have to do with memory? Experimentally, endorphins stimulate growth of the cells in the hippocampus that mediate memory.[23] That explains why exercise training reduces the risk of age-related decline of memory, and additionally, via the 'feel good' factor, has the capacity to reduce depression and is used as antidepressant therapy.

If you can't exercise

So exercise training seems one key step to endorphin-mediated memory improvement. But what about those who cannot or do not wish to exercise? Another way of getting the endorphin stimulus is to travel to Japan, where bathing in 47°C thermal water from Kusatsu increases circulating endorphins. For those who want to follow up this lead, Kusatsu is located in a beautiful national park, not too far from Tokyo. If you can't exercise and can't get to Japan, try sleep, which helps to retain memory. Even a short nap can improve certain aspects of cognitive function. Conversely, sleep deprivation makes memory worse.[2]

Exercising the brain

Practice makes perfect. Does this dictum apply to cognitive function? Cognitive training was given to the subjects of one trial for an initial 5–6 weeks of group training followed about one year later by a booster training period lasting 2–3 weeks.(24) Speed of processing mental activities and the ability to reason both improved, whereas changes in memory were marginal. Overall, mental training helps the brain, just as physical training helps the body. Should you buy Nintendo's Brain Training game? Or play a numbers game such as Sudoku? First principles say that it should help, especially those who do not already do crossword puzzles or play Scrabble or chess.

Diabetes and obesity promote memory loss

Diabetes damages large and small arteries all over the body, and its ravages are well established. The heart, kidneys, eyes, and brain may all suffer, because diabetes promotes heart attacks, kidney failure, poor eyesight, and strokes. More recently another dreaded complication has arisen: mid-life diabetes is associated with cognitive decline.(25) The mechanisms are complex and go beyond increase of high blood pressure and blood cholesterol, to involve damage to the small arteries of the brain. Besides damaging large and small arteries, diabetes lessens the supply of food for the brain, which needs glucose to function well (Fig. 7.8). In the brain, as elsewhere, active insulin is needed for the high rates of transport of glucose into the memory cells of the brain. Conversely, the high blood free fatty acids found in obese diabetics block the uptake of glucose into brain cells.

These fatty acids are totally different from cholesterol. They are released from body fat (technical term: adipose tissue). So why not just get rid of the source of the harmful fatty acids, namely body fat, by a strict diet and test the effect on memory? Indeed, 29 German women with an average body weight of 88 kg had their caloric intake restricted by 30% over three months. In those who lost more than 2% of their body weight, actually not very much, their memory scores improved substantially.(26) Of interest, previous abnormally high insulin levels fell, as did fasting glucose. Blood insulin is usually high in those with diabetes or obesity yet this insulin is not working as it

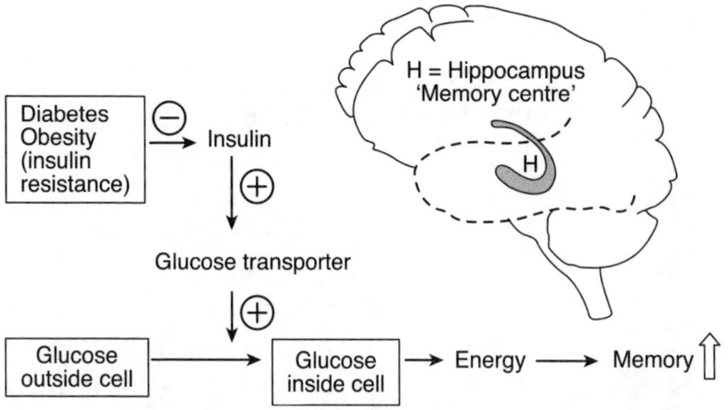

Figure 7.8 Glucose and the memory centre. Brain cells located in the memory centre in the hippocampus (H) require glucose from the blood to be transported into brain cells. For this to happen at optimal rates, the action of the hormone insulin is required. This beneficial action of insulin can be disrupted by conditions that oppose the action of insulin, such as obesity and diabetes, which cause resistance to the glucose-lowering effects of insulin (technical term: insulin resistance). © Opie.

should to decrease blood fatty acids and to promote the metabolism of glucose (Fig. 7.8).

Although this article on caloric restriction in humans was published in one of the very top journals, the results seem too good to be true—can the loss of not much weight, only 2% or somewhat more over three months, really give such memory improvement? If so, was the benefit mediated just by caloric restriction or was it the changes in some metabolic component such as exercise-induced improved sensitivity to insulin and hence better glucose uptake by the brain that did it? Perhaps it was simply a major psychological effect related to the 'feel good' factor associated with successful but modest weight loss?

The Mediterranean diet: can it preserve the mind?

Can food protect the brain? There is a fascinating emerging relationship between the Mediterranean diet and decreased cognitive decline with age (Fig. 7.9). For example, apparently normal New Yorkers of

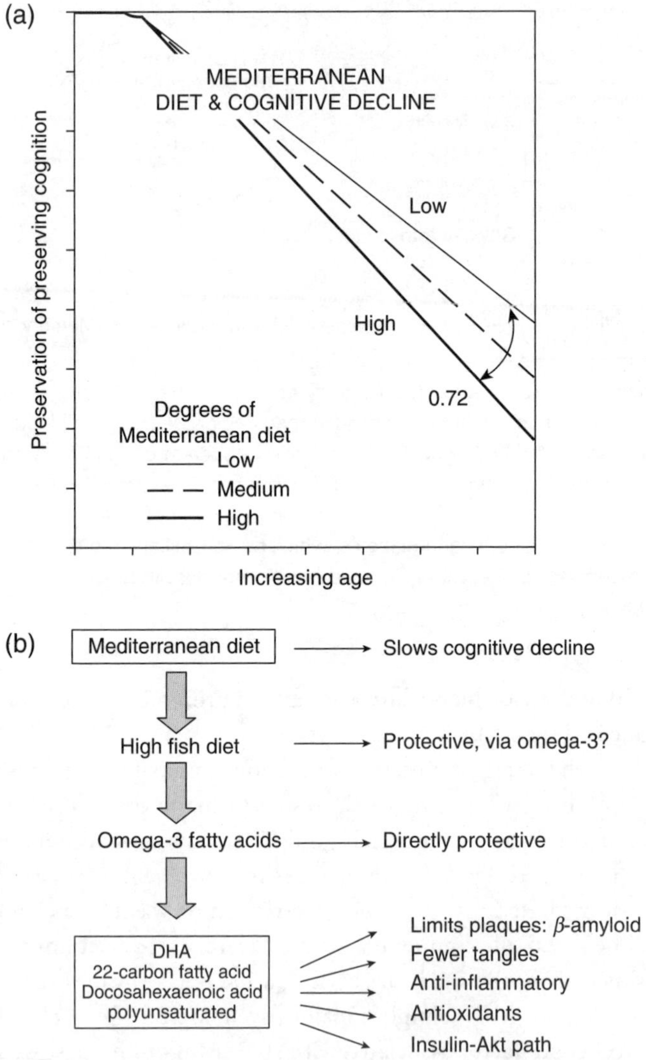

Figure 7.9 The Mediterranean diet mitigates the loss of memory with age.[(27)] High adherence to the diet has a significant reduction (odds ratio, 0.72; 28%) versus low adherence.[(27)] The proposed mechanism is by the high dietary content of omega-3 fatty acids and in particular of DHA (docosahexaenoic acid).[(28)] For mechanisms in detail, see Cole et al. 2009.[(27)]

mean age 77 years eating a highly Mediterranean type of diet had up to 28% less risk of developing cognitive loss.[27] Note that careful scrutiny of the data shows that these imposing percentages reflect relatively small benefits in absolute terms.

What was meant by the Mediterranean diet? As more fully discussed in Chapter 4, pioneering studies from Greece defined this diet as having nine components, five being beneficial (vegetables, legumes, fruit, cereals, and fish), three being detrimental (meat, fat, and fatty dairy products), with the ninth factor being beneficial, namely moderate wine intake. Thus modest protection from cognitive decline adds to the other established benefits of the Mediterranean diet: decreased heart attacks and improved longevity.

The vegetable component

Which of the components of the Mediterranean diet gave the benefit? Plenty of vegetables is one answer according to another American study, this time in Chicago where 3718 citizens were followed for six years.[29] Those who ate 3–4 servings of vegetables every day had about 40% slower decline in memory and related cognitive faculties. Presumably the protective vegetables had all the correct ratios and contents of complex protective substances, some of which we do not yet fully understand.

A word of caution that must be emphasized once again: all these dietary studies are observational (reporting an association), and *do not prove cause-and-effect*. For example, those Americans choosing a Mediterranean diet might have been of one ethnic group rather than another, with different inheritance of Alzheimer's disease, or those already with a healthy lifestyle and superior brains might have been more likely to adopt the Mediterranean diet even before the study began.

A fishy factor

To explain the benefits of the Mediterranean diet, the fish factor is another favourite dietary component. A consistent finding is that those frequently eating fish have better cognition.[30] How much fish? The optimal intake was about 75 grams per day in elderly Norwegian citizens. What is it in the fish that is beneficial? Another study, this time from the

Netherlands, confirmed that fish in the diet, this time more than 20 g per day, delayed cognitive decline in the elderly, and linked fish-eating to an increased intake of long-chain omega-3 fatty acids.(31) The issue of mercury toxicity has been evaluated and largely dismissed in Chapter 4.

Do omega-3 fatty acids improve or protect memory?

The next logical step links higher blood concentrations of omega-3 fatty acids to slower cognitive decline in the elderly.(32) Cognitive decline is age-related and those with higher omega-3 levels behaved as if they were 4–12 years younger. The major gain was in some speed-related activities but there was no change in memory or in fluency of expressing words, so the links between memory and fish oil still remain incomplete. A different issue is the need for omega-3 fatty acids for brain development, as shown in a well-designed study that included brain imaging in young boys.(33)

Folic acid and memory

The word folic comes from the Latin *folium*, meaning leaf. Folic acid is a major component of the leafy vegetables found in the Mediterranean diet. Some argue that folic acid should improve memory because it lowers blood homocysteine levels. Yet a careful analysis of nine studies in the *American Journal of Medicine* (June 2010) failed to show any benefit within three years of treatment. But folic acid was part of the high dose vitamin B mix, with B12 and B6, that helped to counter the brain shrinkage in the elderly.[12]

Drugs and nutritional agents claimed to influence memory

A reduction in acetylcholine-producing brain cells has been implicated in Alzheimer's disease. Logical therapy therefore is to give a drug that inhibits the breakdown of acetylcholine (technical term: anti-cholinesterase). This drug, donepezil or Aricept, delays the rate of deterioration in Alzheimer's disease, being effective over six months but insignificantly so over three years. Nonetheless Aricept is often used with the hope of staving off further deterioration in early Alzheimer's. This drug gave those with only cognitive decline and not true Alzheimer's disease one to two years of protection from developing full-blown Alzheimer's disease but no lasting improvement in memory. Could it delay the eventual onset of age-related memory loss? Unfortunately not, as shown in a careful three-year study reported in the *New England Journal of Medicine.*[34]

Nicotine patches

Nicotine accelerates the release of the neurotransmitter acetylcholine so that the application of nicotine patches often gives memory a short-term boost. Would nicotine patches really help in preventing the transition from memory loss to Alzheimer's? We could find no good study to show that nicotine can delay the onset of Alzheimer's disease in humans. In mice with a genetically-induced model of Alzheimer's disease, chronic nicotine administration decreases the number of amyloid-beta plaques (proposed beneficial effect), while exaggerating the number of tangled fibres (proposed harmful effect).

Smoking

Whereas some early studies suggested that cigarette smoking protects against the development of Alzheimer's disease and that there could be a neuroprotective effect of nicotine, more recent and much larger and better designed studies show that the elderly who smoke and hence inhale nicotine may be at increased rather than decreased risk for serious memory loss. For example, in over 9000 European inhabitants studied for over two years, those who smoked had a higher rate of decline of memory than those who did not. This study, reported in the journal *Neurology* in 2004, was matched by another study on nearly 3500 Japanese-American men living in Honolulu, who were prospectively studied over 4.7 years. Here, smoking in mid-life was associated with a higher risk of late-life memory loss. Thus any direct neuroprotective effect of nicotine (albeit very controversial) is probably more than negated by nicotine-induced damage to blood vessels.

Aspirin and other anti-inflammatories

Population studies suggest that aspirin taken over many years is associated with a lessened risk of Alzheimer's disease by about half, and taking other related anti-inflammatory drugs may have a similar effect. Although these are only observational studies, decreased inflammation is an additional mechanism whereby aspirin could act. This would be logical because one major theory for the full development of Alzheimer's disease is the role of chronic inflammation.[35] Experimentally, proinflammatory messengers (cytokines) are activated by amyloid plaques, thus accelerating the progression of the disease. Although Alzheimer's disease is clearly not only vascular in origin, many factors promoting vascular diseases could worsen the direct adverse effects of Alzheimer's disease.

Aspirin is one of a group of drugs known as the non-steroidal anti-inflammatory drugs (NSAIDs). Of these, ibuprofen (Brufen) is well tested for its effects in retarding the formation of beta-amyloid in animal models of Alzheimer's disease.[36] Hence ibuprofen seems a logical bet as the memory fades in Alzheimer's, albeit not tested in large prospective human trials. Ibuprofen also helps to relieve joint and other skeletal pains. Both aspirin and ibuprofen are contradicted in patients with stomach (peptic) ulcers. Of the other NSAIDs, some modestly accelerate blood vessel disease in humans, so that as a group NSAIDs are not ideal for stalling memory loss.

How solid are the data on aspirin?

So, where do we stand in relation to three important criteria that are required to convincingly prove therapeutic benefit: animal data; human population studies; and prospective controlled human trials? First, animal experiments support the anti-Alzheimer's effects of aspirin and ibuprofen. Second, observational human population studies likewise support the memory-protective role of these agents. But, thirdly and crucially, prospective controlled human studies are either insufficient or missing, so that there is no certainty that these agents can protect from memory loss and Alzheimer's disease. Regarding aspirin, possible but not proven delay of memory loss may be a beneficial side-effect when aspirin is taken for protection against heart attacks or stroke.

Viagra and its friends to the rescue?

As is well known, Viagra (sildenafil) and its friends such as tadalafil (Cialis) and verdenafil (Levitra) promote penile erection by increasing the blood supply. In technical terms, they increase intracellular concentrations of a specific messenger compound (cyclic GMP). This is the same compound that Viagra increases in the human penile blood system. In mice if not in men, Viagra also promotes memory and, furthermore, protects against Alzheimer's disease.(37)

However, there is as yet no evidence that this happy side-effect of Viagra is also found in humans. Of the other two, verdanafil is untested in mice and tadalafil is unlikely to pass the blood-brain barriers to cross into the brain. A better 'brain Viagra' that acts more on the human brain and less elsewhere is in commercial development.

Melatonin

This substance is secreted from the gland at the base of the brain, the pineal gland, in response to darkness. Thus as night falls, so melatonin helps to bring on sleep. Besides its well-known use in countering the awake state of jet lag, it can be used to induce sleep in those Alzheimer's sufferers with its often associated significant sleep disturbances. Melatonin is a powerful antioxidant, and has been tested in rodent models of Alzheimer's disease with conflicting results. There is no dispute about its antioxidant properties in the laboratory. Indeed, one theory of age-related memory loss emphasizes decreased clearance of oxygen free radicals in the brain. However, in most animal experiments the dose of melatonin has been 10 mg per kilo, which translates into about 700–800 mg for a person of average weight. By contrast, the usual human dose is a fraction of the rat or mouse dose, being only 3–10 mg. Thus, the hope that melatonin will save the failing human memory may be vastly exaggerated. Proper human studies are needed.

Tea, stroke prevention, and memory

Green tea is legendary for its supposed health benefits. Experimentally, stroke is reduced by compounds called catechins as found in green but not black tea. By contrast, in population studies drinking either green or black tea, both demonstrated about 20% reduction.(38) Three or more cups per day are protective. The crucial chemical found in both black and green tea is theanine, which protects the inner layer of blood vessels in the brain. Note, however, that there are no prospective long-term studies measuring stroke in which tea is given in comparison say to coffee or to fruit juice, to establish proof-of-concept, so emphasis should be on the more sure ways of stroke reduction such as blood pressure reduction.

Green tea has many fans in Japan where it almost has cult status, and where drinking more of it was associated with less cognitive impairment.(39) But association does not equal causation.

Black tea not green tea is drunk in China, and it too is associated with less cognitive impairment and decline.(40) Maybe the common mechanism to both green and black tea is that both may lessen stroke and by extension, both should reduce memory loss.

Coffee

Regarding coffee, the best and longest study over 28 years found no link between mid-life coffee drinking and late life cognitive performance.(41)

Gingko biloba

This herbal remedy has many benefits ascribed to it, including the hope of countering age-related cognitive loss. In a careful study over a mean of 6.1 years on 3069 participants aged 72 to 96 in six US academic centres, a dose of 120 mg twice daily made no difference at all to the 'normal' rate of cognitive loss.(42)

Hormonal replacement therapy (HRT)

For women and their partners, it is important to know what, if anything, HRT (a combination of oestrogens and progesterone preparations) does to the memory. Although there are certain women who subjectively feel better (and therefore apparently have better memories) when they receive HRT, the sobering fact is that HRT increased stroke by 41% in the large American Women's Health Initiative trial. If major stroke really is increased by this staggering percentage, then small strokes with loss of memory are also likely to be increased. However, the absolute risk of a stroke was small, especially (at a guess) in those with low or normal blood pressures at the start. Women who choose HRT have generally better health and cognitive function before starting than those who do not, hence they also generally end up with better cognitive function. Animal data are also not conclusive; earlier data that rats without ovaries have better memory when given HRT have not been confirmed. In one study, women with Alzheimer's disease who received high doses of oestrogens given by skin patch performed better in memory tests than those who received the placebo.

Testosterone given to the ailing male for the 'andropause' may do many things but there is no evidence that it improves or protects memory. Testosterone medication has several adverse side-effects such as an increased risk of prostatic carcinoma, so it should only be taken under medical supervision.

Logical Alzheimer's theory: attack the plaque?

If the crucial aspect of Alzheimer's is the formation of plaques of amyloid-beta, then logical therapy would be to slow its formation. Such specific therapy is now becoming possible through new drugs that decrease the formation of the precursor amyloid-beta (oligomeric $A\beta_{42}$) molecule that initiates the process of plaque formation.[43] These drugs are the selective amyloid-beta lowering agents (SALA). Tarenflurbil, a drug still under testing, has had promising preliminary results in mild to moderate Alzheimer's disease in that overall function of the patients and their activities of daily living improved by 35–46%, but there was no effect on impaired cognitive function, which is the primary problem.[44]

Once the harmful amyloid-beta plaque is formed, then breaking it down does not seem successful. Indeed, enthusiasm for amyloid-lowering therapy has fallen since the results of therapy with a vaccine that produces antibodies against the amyloid plaques were made public. Decreasing the density of plaques (technical term: 'plaque burden') did not affect cognitive decline.[43] There are several explanations for this failure, including the proposal that the fully formed dense amyloid-beta plaques might be harmless, and their breakdown by the vaccine might produce a more soluble form of the amyloid that could be the real cause of the problem.

Untangling the tangles

The amyloid plaque is only one aspect of the characteristic brain abnormalities found in Alzheimer's disease, the other being the thick tangles of fibres that can strangulate the brain cells. A protein called tau is the major component of these tangles, which can be broken down by a novel drug named, guess what—remberTM. This drug, studied by the University of Aberdeen in Scotland, acts on those parts of the brain critical for memory, where the density of Alzheimer tangles is greatest.(45) In a preliminary trial on 321 patients with mild to moderate Alzheimer's disease, the anti-tangle drug slowed down cognitive decline and improved brain scans. Now a larger trial is underway. Hopefully these and other molecular approaches will eventually result in a simple and specific therapy for Alzheimer's disease.

Even more logical: stop the plaque from forming

American neuroscientists have recently identified a simplified peptide structure, related in part to the structure of the amyloid-beta peptide of Alzheimer's.(46) This peptide was found in mice with a genetic memory defect without any of the typical Alzheimer's changes (i.e. no amyloid plaques or fibrils). Indeed, this same peptide could induce memory defects even in normal rats. Thus, future drug therapy could inhibit the formation of this very early chemical that promotes memory loss.

What if deterioration of memory seriously concerns you?

First, consult Fig. 7.2 and follow it out. Your blood pressure, fasting blood sugar, blood cholesterol, and blood lipid profile patterns (technical term: lipogram) need to be checked and, if abnormal, treated. Rule out small clots travelling from the heart to the brain. These are more common if you have totally irregular heartbeats (atrial fibrillation). Self-check for obesity and lack of exercise (Table 7.1), because weight loss, increased exercise, and cognitive training by mental exercises are important stepping stones to improving memory. While awaiting decisive studies, a wise decision would be to adopt the Mediterranean diet, knowing that it protects the heart and may well protect the brain (Fig. 7.9). Strongly consider high dose omega-3 fatty acids and high dose vitamin B12, B6 and folic acid. If after following these guidelines for 3–6 months there is no improvement, consider consulting a memory loss expert, who may recommend the drug donepezil (Aricept). This works by lessening the rate of breakdown of acetylcholine, one of the neurotransmitters involved in memory.

Summary

Memory is an elusive quality, an important part of what is called cognitive function. These qualities are essential to middle-aged people in order to carry out their professional and personal activities. As more and more people enter the elderly (60–80 years of age) and advanced elderly (80 years and over) age groups, maintenance of memory becomes ever more important in our modern society where self-care has become the norm.

What can be done right now to preserve and protect memory? As the vast majority of elderly people have problems with relatively minor though increasing degrees of cognitive loss, keeping the arteries open and the brain tissue healthy is the best way to go. That means control of blood pressure and cholesterol together with a Mediterranean diet and exercise, even though these measures are not yet fully established. In brief, what is good for the heart is also good for the brain.

A major but small new study showed that high doses of vitamins B12, B6 and folic acid could slow the brain shrinkage found in the elderly even with only mild cognitive loss.

Much more specifically, molecular therapy designed to specifically target the formation and breakdown of harmful beta-amyloid plaques is under clinical trial testing in advanced to moderate Alzheimer's disease with, so far, mixed results. More promising therapy is aimed at breaking down the fibre tangles that are also involved. Another tip for the future: watch for the 'Brain Viagra'.

Chapter 8

The Heart-Mind Connection

Traditionally, there have been two somewhat opposing ways of looking at the effect of the mind on the heart and vice versa. First, there is the way of inner peace and calm, almost detaching the mind from the body, as epitomized by the traditional religions of Asia. For example, in the opening line of David Guterson's book, *Snow Falling on Cedars*, an Asiatic man '*sat proudly upright, his palms placed softly on the table. The posture of a man who had detached himself insofar as this is possible.*' By contrast, the modern Westerner is very aware of mind-body interactions, for example often linking psychological stress to heart disease.

Heart attacks were once commonly linked to the well-known A-type personality, first described in the 1970s, and characterized by those who are always agitated, anxious, angry, impulsive, irritable, competitive, depressed, and dissatisfied. Since then, detailed studies have failed to find clear links between type A personality and heart attacks, so that the emphasis on personality traits has largely faded away. Conversely, it is now clear that acute psychological stress can precipitate a heart attack, but especially in those already made to be coronary-prone by other major risk factors.(1) This makes sense because such acute stress will put the body's emergency systems on 'high alert', ready for fight or flight, and for psychological fright. Rapid activation of the adrenaline system increases heart rate and blood pressure (BP) (Fig. 1.2), with greater demand for oxygen by the heart muscle. In the presence of existing coronary artery disease, it is easy to see how a heart attack could be provoked.

If stress provokes heart attacks and raises the blood pressure, then stress reduction should protect the heart. This chapter considers the role of stress modification by mindfulness and meditation, followed by the role of stress reduction in medical diseases such as hypertension and heart attacks. We shall consider these three M's: Mindfulness, Meditation, and their Medical application.

Mindfulness

As the word 'mind' has many meanings, so does mindfulness. One modern version is the cultivation of a state in which bodily needs are temporarily set aside to allow the mind to dominate. Another is 'focusing attention in a non-judgemental way or accepting on the experience occurring in the present moment'.[2]

These are difficult concepts that are differently propounded by different experts. A very recent long and complex article in the *Annals of the New York Academy of Sciences*[3] argues that current views of mindfulness have deviated significantly from the roots of this state of mind, which go back to ancient Buddhist teaching. Even that apparently goes further back to the original Indian Theravadin tradition, especially a text called the *Mahasatipathana Sutta*: Mindfulness Immersed in the Body. Of interest, Buddhism was born out of Hinduism round about the 5th century BCE. There is still some overlap, especially in relation to control of the body by the mind—just witness the Hindu devotees who sit in strange postures outside temples for days and weeks on end.

Mindfulness and breathing

In the practice of these early Tibetan Buddhist and Indian versions, the initial phase of mindfulness starts by focusing on the target object to the exclusion of all other objects and experiences. But what is the target object? The classical Buddhist teaching is to focus on breathing in and out and while being peripherally aware of the body as one breathes. Buddhist concepts of emptiness and enlightenment may seem beyond the scientific field of enquiry, although we know that repeated deep breathing in ordinary people can produce hyperventilation, which induces tingling of the hands and feet and dizziness of the brain. These changes working on the contemplative brain may contribute what is called 'mindfulness'.

How can mindfulness be developed? This aim is complex and not for all, nor is the need to develop mindfulness as readily apparent to the Western mind as it is obvious to the Asian mind. 'The four foundations of the classical Buddhist tradition are bodily sensations, feelings, thoughts, and mental contents'.[3] The aim of focusing on deep breathing is to allow the moment to moment experience of the thoughts, sensations, and pictures that enter the mind to be in a 'bare' format, stripped of any associated emotional reactions. In that state, different positive and negative thoughts enter and leave the mind. In the terminology used, the positive thoughts are called 'adaptive' and the negative thoughts 'maladaptive'. Repetitive training facilitates adaptive and decreases maladaptive thoughts, feelings, and behaviour.

A modern view

Harvard Women's Health Watch wrote in 2004 that mindfulness is the ability to pay attention to what you are experiencing from moment to moment while excluding thoughts about the past and concerns about the future. Mindfulness is proposed as a state that can increase enjoyment of life, expand the capacity to cope with illness, and reduce stress. This American view is fully compatible with the contemplative view of life provided by Buddhism. As we shall see, mindfulness can be enhanced by meditation.

Meditation

Meditation in Latin simply means 'contemplation', which stretches all the way from the simple to the complex. In simple terms, contemplating the wonders of nature can induce meditation. In a more complex sense, meditation is disciplined, self-searching, self-criticizing. In religious and personal terms, it includes prayer, asking for forgiveness, and through meditation achieving an insight into personal weak and strong points. By meditation inner conflicts can be resolved. The concept of inner peace actually stretches from the Buddhist view across religions (I think of the interior of the Blue Mosque in Istanbul, or Westminster Abbey when there are no other visitors, or the quiet beauty within Vézelay Abbey in central France. You may picture any other impressive and quiet religious building that you might have experienced.) In my view, all forms of contemplative meditation can stimulate the vagus nerves of the autonomic nervous system to reduce heart rate and blood pressure (see also Fig 1.3).

Other routes to enhanced vagal stimulation

Thus meditation unexpectedly uses the same mechanism, vagal stimulation, as does exercise training to slow the resting heart rate and drop the blood pressure (Fig. 8.1). Thus, in contrast to physically inactive mindfulness, increased physical activity is another totally different way of promoting vagal activity and indirectly decreasing the blood pressure at rest. Furthermore, the vagal messenger, acetylcholine, is important for memory formation in the brain so that, very speculatively, meditation could enhance memory.

Nirvana means 'extinction' in Sanskrit

For the Buddhist, meditation is a specific term that includes the achieving of a state of self-awareness and inner calm called nirvana, the state of mental freedom and 'extinction' of the body achieved by excluding desire and surmounting individual consciousness. Theravada Buddhism conceives of nirvana as tranquillity and

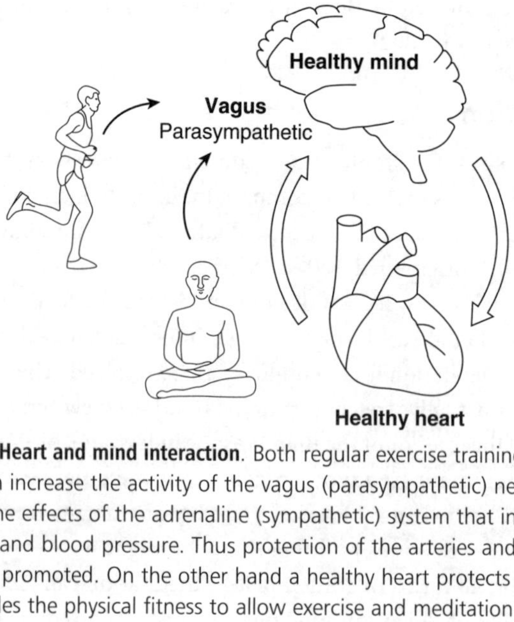

Figure 8.1 Heart and mind interaction. Both regular exercise training and meditation increase the activity of the vagus (parasympathetic) nerve that opposes the effects of the adrenaline (sympathetic) system that increases heart rate and blood pressure. Thus protection of the arteries and heart health are promoted. On the other hand a healthy heart protects the brain and provides the physical fitness to allow exercise and meditation.

peace; Mahayana Buddhism equates it with sunyata (emptiness), dharma-kaya (the essence of the Buddha), and dharma-datu (ultimate reality).

Yoga

In its Indian form yoga is closely related to achieving nirvana. Yoga is a mind-body exercise that combines stretching and controlled breathing to achieve relaxation and a stabilized mood. Yoga uses breathing techniques, exercise, and meditation with the aims of improving health and happiness. A current American craze is naked yoga, which if co-ed seems less likely to achieve any relaxation.

Transcendental meditation

This mind-body meditation programme is derived from the ancient Indian Vedic tradition, with the aim of engendering a state of 'restful alertness' that is aimed at detaching oneself from stress by silent meditation and retention of a mantra. This state may be physically promoted by sitting comfortably with closed eyes and a slower rate of breathing. The result is reduced blood pressure and heart rate.[(4)] Of note, training in this technique improves mindfulness,[(2)] and emerging studies suggest medical application (see following section).

Religious faith

Studies on devout Catholics and other religious groups point to a number of associated benefits: a better psychological state after stroke, better coping with medical illnesses in the elderly even during terminal illness, and 32% lesser risk of mortality in those who have regularly attended church.[(5)] Mere outer observance is insufficient—that is called religiosity.[(6)] There should be inner commitment. Of course it is very difficult to find studies that would convince the medical scientist of the benefits of prayer, because of the difficulty of sorting out the many factors that may be involved and the impossibility of doing a randomized study. Is it just the association of faith with a certain personality type that in any case would give protection from bodily disease, or is it the act of prayer and the inner peace that comes with it? Which is decisive?

Medical application

Does stress relief reduce blood pressure?

Clearly meditation, whether achieved by yoga, Buddhist or transcendental meditation, or by contemplative prayer, can reduce psychological stress, which in turn reduces the blood pressure in the short term, but can it help in the therapy of sustained BP elevation? There are several conflicting studies, but very few are well designed.[7] The review that merits most credibility, meeting the stringent standards of the UK-based Cochrane review group, found only a small non-significant reduction of blood pressure. In their 71-page report, the authors also found that most of the studies that they could review were poorly designed without scientific finesse.[8] Fifteen studies had to be excluded because the people involved had normal BPs to start with (dropping the BP in such people is not the same as decreasing it in those whose BP is continuously and abnormally sustained).

Provoked temporary stress and stress relief were used in a small but very interesting study just published by the American Heart Association.[9] Stress management was achieved by self-repetition of phrases that focused on feelings of bodily heaviness, calm, and warmth in large muscles. This procedure lessened the BP rise during mental stress, during which the heart rate also decreased compared with controls. Measurements with the electrocardiogram (ECG) showed increased vagal tone and a small but significantly dampened BP response to stress including measurements over 24 hours.[9]

Group transcendental meditation and blood pressure

The effects of transcendental meditation on BP were tested in another well-designed study.[4] Transcendental meditation was practised twice daily for periods of 20 minutes for three months, after an introductory seven-step course. Transcendental meditation was then given to small groups of university students 'at risk of hypertension' by being overweight but with initially normal BPs (mean values of 122/79 mmHg; very close to normal values of 120/80 mmHg). Transcendental meditation dropped their BP by 5/3 mmHg on average. That is about the level of BP reduction achieved with only one BP-reducing agent in those with elevated blood pressures. Experience from another much longer and larger study shows that modest elevations of BP within the high normal range can safely be reduced by a single BP-lowering agent (in this case a drug called candesartan) but that the BP creeps back when the therapy stops. My guess is that for transcendental meditation to have a long-term effect it would also have to be sustained over many years at some significant cost of time and money but with a beneficial side-effect of fewer stress-related psychological symptoms.

Transcendental meditation and relaxation therapy vs BP tablets

For many with high blood pressure the drug therapy of hypertension is now so simple and essentially without side-effects that the convenience of one or two daily tablets far outstrips the time-requiring benefits of meditation and relaxation therapy. Furthermore there is no long-term well-designed study to show that stress reduction or group transcendental meditation reduces the blood pressure in those with true hypertension. For those whose prime wish is wish to develop inner peace by transcendental meditation or yoga, even a small fall in blood pressure would be a bonus. In some, I suspect, the fall in blood pressure would be larger than in others.

Effects of transcendental meditation on vascular disease

Transcendental meditation, by promoting relaxation, should decrease the blood pressure and hence stroke, as is being investigated in an ongoing long-term study funded by the National Institutes of Health of the USA. In the meantime, we already have a pointer in the positive direction because transcendental meditation modestly lessens disease of the large carotid arteries that supply blood to the brain.[10]

For the medical scientist, properly designed studies are required to test accurately the effects of several different types of meditation and yoga in those people with modestly elevated blood pressures. This is a considerable challenge because of the different disciplines that would have to be rigorously brought into the trial design: psychology, exercise physiology, hypertension, and statistics. A similar problem of poorly designed studies without proof of concept extends to patients with anxiety disorder. Common sense but no solid scientific data says that severe anxiety should respond to meditation-based stress management.

Stress and heart attacks

Let's look at the big picture. We probably all know of someone who under major stress had a heart attack—but how often does that happen? Large population studies tell us more about the incidence. The INTERHEART study provides the best information we have of about 25 000 people with previous heart attacks. It was a worldwide study covering 52 countries, as discussed in Chapter 3. In this definitive study psychological stress was a newly-confirmed risk factor[(1)]—but was only one of nine factors. Three of the nine factors were protective—namely exercise, alcohol, and a diet high in fruit and vegetables—and there were six adverse factors, namely smoking, diabetes, hypertension, abdominal obesity, the blood cholesterol pattern, and psychological factors.

If all six adverse factors were equally important, which is roughly true, then each would account for about 17% of heart attacks, including psychological factors of which the two major problems were acute stress at home or at work, and depression.[(1)] The exact contribution of psychological factors varied between ethnic groups, being more common both in Chinese (including those living in Hong Kong) and in Latin American people than in others.

Depression and future heart attacks

Another large population study was very different—looking into the future and asking whether those with certain psychological features would be more prone to the future development of heart attacks or angina. In this equally huge study, the Whitehall II study, 10 308 British civil servants working in London, England, were followed for 12 years. At the start they had to be free of coronary disease (heart attacks or angina) and the follow-up was for 12 years. There was a 33% increase in the development of new heart attacks or angina in those chronically 'feeling low'. This psychological state, commonly called depression, included 'distress, discomfort, dissatisfaction, and feelings of hopelessness over time and regardless of the situation'.[(11)]

Unexpected links between stress or depression and heart attacks

Poor lifestyle choices may explain the link between stress, depression, and other psychological problems and increased cardiovascular risk.(12) Dr Hamer and co-workers from University College London used data from the Scottish Health Survey to measure psychological distress and behavioural and pathophysiological risk factors for heart attacks and stroke in 6576 men and women followed for about seven years. They asked about general levels of happiness, experience of depression and anxiety, and sleep disturbances. Those psychologically distressed had a 54% increased risk of cardiovascular events. They also had poor lifestyle choices such as increased smoking and decreased physical activity. Note that a poor socioeconomic status predisposes both to depression and to ignorance of the risks for heart attacks, and we should also take note of the inability of depressed people to be aware of the early symptoms of heart disease.

Beneficial vs harmful stress

Stress is not always distress. We have all had the experience at school and probably at university of preparation for examinations causing stress as a positive factor in getting all the revision done, provided that we had been working consistently throughout the academic year. Conversely, in those not prepared, the stress of examinations is huge. And then there are those who even if fully prepared are still overwhelmed by emotions that cause marked fear-engendering stress. The links between heart disease and stress lie in the emotions that cannot be contained or easily dealt with—sometimes acute, sometimes sustained. Practising mindfulness and other inner resources as described in this chapter builds up emotional strength, making us more ready to counterbalance unexpected severe stresses in the future.

Bottom line

Stress is one of six factors identified in a large multinational study as promoting heart attacks. Even if there is no proof that treatment of stress lessens the chance of future heart attacks, common sense says that stress in a person with prior stress-associated heart symptoms merits therapy in its own right. Even for people suffering from substantial psychological stress, there are usually other risk factors for heart disease that must be put right.

Likewise significant sustained depression calls for medication and psychotherapy. Stress assails all of us from time to time so let's learn more about how to deal with it.

How to deal with psychological stress

Practical pragmatic policy

It is very hard to alter one's inherent personality, one's outlook on life, and one's inner philosophy, or to change fundamentally one's reaction to stress. It is much easier to alter externals. Look at the experience of the New York stockbrokers receiving medication for high blood pressure (Chapter 6). They simply kept on with the same stressed pattern of life, except that they each bought a dog and were therefore forced to take exercise and to interact with their dog, with the result that their blood pressure came under control. Probably the dog also brought greater inherent stability or, in psychological parlance, increased the positive affect of the stockbrokers. This type of change is feasible, desirable, and practical.

For those who exercise regularly, psychological stress is often effectively countered by vigorous exercise such as a gym workout. For others, religious meditation and prayer give reassurance and meaning to life. Such devotion can increase a certain type of mindfulness called spirituality (a mind that is not concerned with the material). For still others, the answer lies in stress relief by the yoga mat or by transcendental meditation. Or contact with nature by nurturing a garden or even pot plants can be constructive and relaxing.

Personally, I meditate and exercise simultaneously by walking in the greenery of Newlands Forest on the slopes of Table Mountain, near to our home. I also try to develop focused meditation when in our garden, where looking at flowers and plants and trees relaxes me, and then actively let my mind wander through various problems while working out how to deal with them. But I also believe that regular intense exercise promotes cardioprotective vagal activity and I start the day early with many lengths of an Olympic-sized pool. In the end, it comes down to personal choices between several ways of recognizing the importance of stress and its relief in life.

Changing personality versus changing lifestyle

The type A person, tense and very focused, contrasts with the type B person who has inner calmness, happiness, and a balanced attitude—the type of person that hypothetically is a role model for society—as well as with several other personalities, namely types C, D, and even E. Should we not stop worrying about the difficult and nearly impossible task of trying to change our personalities and fix on the externals that can be changed? The basic rules remain: non-smoking, ideal body weight, daily exercise, healthy diet, and moderate alcohol (Table 3.1). Of these, moderate alcohol is the least protective and, thus, the least essential. This lifestyle will give maximal protection from heart attacks and stroke.

The healthy heart leads to the healthy mind

Knowing that there is protection from heart attack and stroke by following these five simple steps feeds back to inner peace of mind. The simple message is, if you do what you can, you will be rewarded. That knowledge creates a reassuring inner self, irrespective of the basic type of personality. Additional 'inner peace' depends on individual choice. Although religion should help develop inner peace and calm, today there is, unfortunately, a link between over-dogmatic organized religion and violence, even extending to terrorism. Nonetheless, on an individual basis a reflective religious approach can generate extra calm and extra capacity to deal with life and, particularly, with interpersonal problems. For some, significant religion means daily devotion; for others it means a retreat to a secluded group in India or Japan or even to a monastery or convent. For me, those precious privileged years at Oxford were a shelter from the tough outside world while building up inner resources.

Does a healthy mind lead to a healthy heart?

Common sense says yes—but what are the facts? Many of the aspects of mindfulness and meditation leading to a relaxed or detached mental attitude will, like physical exercise, increase the activity of that part of the silent ('autonomic') nervous system that slows the heart and drops the blood pressure. As already described (Figs. 1.3 and 6.1) this vagal system balances the opposing activating sympathetic system that increases heart rate and blood pressure. Thus, mindfulness and meditation by reducing heart rate and blood pressure should reduce the risk of heart attacks. Unfortunately there have been few if any well-designed scientific studies to support these common-sense proposals.

Passion and play as active meditation

Many of the approaches here explored are aimed at dampening excess stress, promoting inner peace and the contemplative life. But what about passion? There are many kinds of passion, for example the passion of the artist, that of the scientist aiming to push knowledge to the limits, that of the medical missionary, and of course the sometimes evanescent passion of love.

The word 'passion' is derived from the Old French for 'suffering', but now has at least seven meanings, at least in France according to a standard French dictionary. Two of those are directly relevant: first, emotional or intellectual activities that dominate life through the intensity of their consequences; and the enthusiasm of an artist for creative work. People with such passions are already communicating with their inner selves. Such life-giving passion is what could be called active meditation, the opposite to emptying the mind and waiting to see what then fills it.

Play is another form of active meditation. This word is derived from the Old English, to exercise. Regarding play, listen to George Vaillant, Professor of Psychiatry at Harvard Medical School.[13] He looks at retirement happiness—the inevitable time when many professionals have to face their inner and outer selves. Besides a sense of purpose and a good marriage, the most important key in his studies was learning 'how to play again', in other words exercising the mind and opening up to the new. He defines play as those patterns of behaviour highly satisfying to the individual without damaging others, without significant monetary reward, and often a response to a new inner self that does not necessarily seek the approval or encouragement of society.

Thus to play in this sense is to renew the mind and actively to explore the outside emotional world.

Conclusion

The heart-body-mind inter-relationships remain complex. Overall happiness and overall good health go closely together, but we know that good physical health can be achieved by key lifestyle changes (Chapter 3) and by pharmacological medication, yet without the necessity for any in-depth personality changes. In addition, increased mindfulness and meditation can help to relieve stress to maintain the mind-body balance, especially when combined with lifestyle modification. Herewith my final reminder of the ideal five-point protective lifestyle: non-smoking, ideal body weight, ideal diet, daily exercise, and last and probably least important, moderate alcohol (my personal choice for the latter is a fine Pinot Noir).

References

References: Chapter 2

1. Ross, R. New Engl J Med 1999; 340: 115.
2. Yusuf, S et al. Lancet 2004; 364: 937.
3. Bibbins-Domingo, K et al. New Engl J Med 2010; 362: 590.

References: Chapter 3

1. Chiuve SE, et al. Circulation 2006; 114: 160.
2. Chiuve SE, et al. Circulation 2008; 118: 947.
3. Dam van RM, et al. Br Med J 2008; 337: a1440.
4. Kvaavik E, et al. Arch Intern Med 2010;170: 711.
5. Knoops KTB, et al. JAMA 2004; 292: 1433.
6. Keys A, Keys N. How to Eat Well and to Stay Well. The Mediterranean Way. Doubleday, 1975.
7. Mitrou PN, et al. Arch Intern Med 2007; 167: 2461.
8. Di Castelnuovo A, et al. Arch Intern Med 2006; 166: 2437.
9. Hines LM, et al. N Engl J Med 2001; 344: 549.
10. Beulens JWJ, et al. Atherosclerosis 2010; 212: 281.
11. Opie LH, Lecour S. Eur Heart J 2007; 28: 1683.
12. Demrow HS, et al. Circulation 1995; 91: 1182.
13. Karatzi KN, et al. Am J Hypertens 2005; 18: 1161.
14. Ducimetiere P. Dialogues in Cardiovascular Medicine 2008; 13: 193; see www.dialogues-cvm.org.
15. Gaziano TA, et al. Lancet 2008; 371: 923.
16. Sheleson SE, et al. J Clin Invest 2006; 116: 1793.
17. Ridker PM, et al. New Engl J Med 2008: 359; 2195.
18. Chow CK, et al. Circulation 2010; 121: 750.
19. Leupker RV, et al. Circulation 2010; 121: 1280.
20. Kivimaki M, et al. Lancet 2008; 372: 1648.
21. Diabetes Prevention Program Research Group. Lancet 2009; 374: 1677.

References: Chapter 4

1. Shai I, et al. N Engl J Med 2008; 359: 229.
2. de Lorgeril M, et al. Circulation 1999; 99: 779.
3. Barzi F, et al. Eur J Clin Nutr 2003; 57: 604.

4. Estruch R, et al. Annal Intern Med 2006; 145: 1.
5. Teres S, et al. PNAS 2008; 105: 13811.
6. Salas-Salvado J, et al. Arch Intern Med 2008; 168: 2449.
7. Martínez-González MA, et al. BMJ 2008; 336: 1348.
8. Samaha A, et al. New Engl J Med 2003; 348: 2074.
9. Halton TL, et al. New Engl J Med 2006; 155: 1991.
10. Sacks FM, et al. N Engl J Med 2009; 360: 859.
11. Barclay AW, et al. Am J Clin Nutr 2008; 87: 627.
12. Jenkins DJ. JAMA 2008; 300: 2742.
13. Esposito K, et al. Ann Intern Med 2009; 151: 306.
14. Fung TT, et al. Arch Intern Med 2008; 168: 713.
15. Ford AL, et al. BMJ 2010; 340: b5388 doi:10.1136/bmj.b5388.
16. Harris WS, et al. Circulation 2009; 119: 902.

References: Chapter 5

1. Bjelakovic G, et al. JAMA 2007; 297: 842.
2. Lonn E, et al. JAMA 2005; 293: 1338.
3. Miller ER 3rd, et al. Ann Int Med 2005; 142: 37.
4. Podmore ID, et al. Nature 1998; 392: 559.
5. Pitsavos C, et al. Am J Clin Nutr 2005; 82: 694.
6. Christen S, et al. Proc Nat Acad Sci 1997; 94: 3217.
7. Hollenberg NK, et al. Circulation 2007; 116: 2360.
8. Taubert D, et al. JAMA 2007; 298: 49.
9. Lange H, et al. New Engl J Med 2004; 350: 2673.
10. Rodionov RN, et al. Arterioscler Thromb Vasc Biol 2008; 28: 1031.
11. Loscalzo J. N Engl J Med 2006; 354: 1629.
12. Lee M, et al. Stroke 2010; 41: 932.
13. Saposnik G, et al. Stroke 2009; 40: 1365.
14. Sesso HD, et al. JAMA 2008; 300: 2123.
15. Gaziano JM, et al. JAMA 2009; 301: 52.
16. HealthDay @ www.businessweek.com/print/lifestyle/content/healthday/638197.html. Accessed 24 April, 2010.
17. Palmer JR, et al. Arch Intern Med 2008; 168: 1487.
18. Tunnicliffe JM, et al. Appl Physiol Nutr Metab 2008; 33: 1301.
19. Lopez-Garcia E, et al. Ann Intern Med 2008; 148: 904.
20. van Gelder BM, et al. Eur J Clin Nutr 2007; 61: 22618.
21. Lopez-Garcia E, et al. Circulation 2006; 113: 2045.
22. Reid IR, et al. Arch Intern Med 2008; 168: 2276.
23. Jackson R, et al. New Engl J Med 2006; 354: 7669.
24. Kontogianni MD, et al. Nutrition 2009; 25: 165.
25. Rossouw JE, et al. Arch Intern Med 2008; 168: 2245.

References: Chapter 6

1. Eisenberg L. Br J Psychiat 1986; 148: 497.
2. St Clair Gibson A, Noakes TD. Brit J Sports Med 2004; 38: 797.
3. Truelson T, et al. Stroke 2003; 34: 856.
4. Surtees PG, et al. Neurology 2008; 70: 788.
5. Allen K, et al. Hypertension 2001; 38: 815.
6. Hamer M, et al. J Am Coll Cardiol 2008; 52: 2156.
7. Gruber AJ, et al. PLoS ONE 2009; 4(4): e5062. doi:10.1371/journal.pone0.0005062.
8. Volkow ND. JAMA 2009; 301: 1148.

References: Chapter 7

1. Cao X, et al. Europ J Neurosci 2007; 25: 1815.
2. Walker MP. Harvard Rev Psychiatry 2008; 16: 287.
3. Solms M, Turnbull O. The Brain and the Inner World. Other Press, 2002.
4. Li F, et al. New Engl J Med 2009; 361: 302.
5. Querfurth HW, et al. New Engl J Med 2010; 362: 329.
6. Andreassen NC. Brave New Brain. Oxford University Press, 2001, p138, p263.
7. Strassburger TJ. Stroke 1997; 28: 1410.
8. Blennow K, et al. Lancet 2006; 368: 387.
9. Holtzman JL, et al. Lancet 2008; 372: 1381.
10. Drachman DA, et al. Neurology 2006; 67: 1340.
11. Smith AD. Dispelling Myths about Alzheimer's Disease. Oxford Medicine, 2009, p1–2.
12. Smith AD, et al. Plos One 2010; 5: e12244.
13. Devanand DP, et al. Arch Neurol 2005; 62: 975.
14. Hillman CH, et al. Nat Rev Neurosci 2008; 9: 58.
15. Larson EB, et al. Ann Intern Med 2006; 144: 73.
16. Eggermont LH, et al. J Am Geriatr Soc 2009; 57: 1750.
17. Hillman CH, et al. Nat Rev Neurosci 2008; 9: 58.
18. Berchtold NC, et al. Neuroscience 2005; 133: 853.
19. Molteni R, et al. Neuroscience 2002; 112: 803.
20. Lautenschlager NT, et al. JAMA 2008; 300: 1027.
21. Liu-Ambrose T, et al. Arch Intern Med 2010; 170:170.
22. Bender T, et al. Eur J Appl Physiol 2007; 100: 371.
23. Koehl M, et al. FASEB J 2008; 22: 2253.
24. Ball K, et al. JAMA 2002; 288: 2271.
25. Biessels GJ, et al. Lancet Neurol 2008; 7: 184.
26. Witte AV, et al. Proc Natl Acad Sci USA 2009; 106: 1255.
27. Scarmeas N, et al. Arch Neurol 2009; 66: 216.
28. Cole GM, et al. Prostaglandins Leukot Essent Fatty Acids 2009; 81: 213.

29. Morris MC, et al. Neurology 2006; 67: 1370.
30. Nurk E, et al. Am J Clin Nutr 2007; 86: 1470.
31. van Gelder BM, et al. Am J Clin Nutr 2007; 85: 1142.
32. Dullemeijer C, et al. Am J Clin Nutr 2007; 86: 1479.
33. McNamara RHK, et al. Am J Clin Nutrition 2010; 91(4): 1060.
34. Peteresen RC, et al. NEJM 2005; 352: 2379.
35. Etminan M, et al. BMJ 2003; 327: 128.
36. Heneka MT. Brain 2005; 128: 1442.
37. Puzzo D, et al. J Neurosci 2009; 29: 8075.
38. Arab L, et al. Stroke 2009; 40: 1786.
39. Kuriyama S. Am J Clin Nutr 2006; 83: 355.
40. Ng TP, et al. Am J Clin Nutr 2008; 88: 224.
41. Laitala VS, et al. Am J Clin Nutr 2009; 90: 640.
42. Snitz BE, et al. JAMA 2009; 302: 2663.
43. Holmes C, et al. Lancet 2008; 372: 216.
44. Wilcock GK, et al. Lancet Neurology 2008; 7: 483.
45. Wischik C. University of Aberdeen press release, 29 July 2008; accessed 14.11.2008.
46. Lesne S, et al. Nature 2006; 440: 352.

References: Chapter 8

1. Rosengren A, et al. Lancet 2004; 364: 953.
2. Tanner MA, et al. J Clin Psychol 2009; 65: 574.
3. Rapgay L, et al. Ann N Y Acad Sci 2009; 1172: 148.
4. Nidich SI, et al. Am J Hypertens 2009; 22: 1326.
5. Giaquinto S, et al. Stroke 2007; 38: 993.
6. Feinstein M, et al. Circulation 2010; 121: 659.
7. Canter PH. BMJ 2003; 326: 1049.
8. Dickinson HO, et al. Cochrane Database Syst Rev 2008; 23: CD004935.
9. Nolan RP, et al. Hypertension 2010; 55: 1033.
10. Castillo-Richmond A, et al. Stroke 2000; 31: 568.
11. Nabi H, et al. BMJ 2008; 337: a118.
12. Hamer M, et al. J Am Coll Cardiol 2008; 52: 2156.
13. Vaillant GE, et al. Am J Psychiat. 2006; 163: 682.

Index

Note: page numbers in *italics* refer to Figures and Tables.

Good Health Care - The Big 5 (31)

BMI - (45)

Warning Indicators of Impending Heart Disease (The Big 5) (54

BP ↑; HDL/LDL ↕; Blood Glucose ↑; Ultra-sensitive C-reactive protein

Diet - Mediterranean (58)

Add Omega-3 capsules (79) (85 1,000 mg a day

Less cheese

Stomach "Feeling full" - 20 minute delay (75)

Avocados (80)

Water (107) (Tap better than bottled

Coffee (108) → (Memory Loss ↓?)

(To Do (1) Read Mind over Matter (113 ff

(2) Memory (Ch 7)

(Aspirin - 163)

(3) Emotions/Stress (Ch 8)